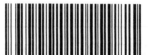

Medicine Pocketbook

From the publishers of the *Tarascon Pocket Pharmacopoeia*

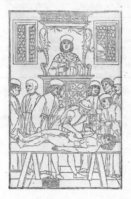

Joseph Esherick, MD, FAAFP
Departments of Family Medicine and Inpatient Medicine
Ventura County Medical Center
Clinical Asst. Prof. of Family Medicine
UCLA School of Medicine

JONES & BARTLETT
LEARNING

World Headquarters
Jones & Bartlett Learning
5 Wall Street
Burlington, MA 01803
978-443-5000
info@jblearning.com
www.jblearning.com

Jones and Bartlett's books and products are available through most bookstores and online booksellers. To contact Jones & Bartlett Learning directly, call 800-832-0034, fax 978-443-8000, or visit our website, www.jblearning.com.

Production Credits
Publisher: Christopher Davis
Senior Acquisitions Editor: Nancy Anastasi Duffy
Senior Editorial Assistant: Jessica Acox
Supervising Production Editor: Daniel Stone
Production Editor: Katherine Crighton
Associate Production Editor: Melissa Elmore
Senior Marketing Manager: Barb Bartoszek
V.P., Manufacturing and Inventory Control: Therese Connell
Composition: Toppan Best-set Premedia Limited
Cover Design: Kristin E. Parker
Cover Image: Courtesy of the National Library of Medicine
Printing and Binding: Cenveo
Cover Printing: Cenveo

ISBN-13: 9781284084023
6048
Printed in the United States of America
17   10

DEDICATION

I would like to dedicate this book to my parents, my wife Gina, and my daughter Sophia. This project would not have been completed without your unending support.

CONTENTS

REVIEWERS

Theresa Cho, MD
Family Medicine

Daniel Clark, MD, FACC, FAHA
Cardiology

Robert Deamer, PharmD, BCPS
Clinical Pharmacist

Robert Dergalust, MD
Neurology

Lauren G. Ficks, MD
Endocrinology

David Fishman, MD
Internal Medicine, Critical Care,
Anesthesia

Saumil Gandhi, MD
Nephrology

James J. Helmer, Jr., MD
Family Medicine, Geriatric Medicine

Mark Lepore, MD
Family Medicine, Hospitalist

Charles Menz, MD
Gastroenterology

Duane Pearson, MD
Rheumatology

Stephanus Philip, MD
Internal Medicine

John G. Prichard, MD
Family Medicine

Javier Romero, MD, FACS
General Surgery, Critical Care

Rick Rutherford, MD
Family Medicine

Gail Simpson, MD, FACP
Infectious Disease

Evan Slater, MD
Hematology-Oncology

George Yu, MD, FACP, FCCP
Pulmonology and Sleep Disorders

PREFACE

The **Tarascon Hospital Medicine Pocketbook** is an evidence-based, point-of-care reference for the busy clinician or student to use on the hospital wards or in the ICU. This pocket reference provides inpatient clinicians with critical information about the evaluation and management of every common medical disorder encountered in the hospital, including the most common conditions encountered in the ICU. This pocketbook is packed with tables and algorithms intended to quickly direct the busy clinician to an evidence-based approach to manage all medical problems encountered in the hospital.

The **Tarascon Hospital Medicine Pocketbook** is an essential guide for all practicing hospitalists, medical students, resident physicians and midlevel providers who work in the hospital setting.

I would like to thank all my colleagues who have passed on to me countless clinical pearls, most of which I have incorporated into this pocketbook. I would also like to thank the hospital librarian, Janet Parker, who has worked so hard to acquire virtually all of the reference articles that were used for the preparation of this manuscript.

The information within this pocketbook has been compiled from sources believed to be reliable. Nevertheless, the **Tarascon Hospital Medicine Pocketbook** is intended to be a clinical guide only; it is not meant to be a replacement for sound clinical judgment. Although painstaking efforts have been made to find all errors and omissions, some errors may remain. If you find an error or wish to make a suggestion, please email your comments to editor@tarascon.com

Best wishes,

Joe Esherick, MD, FAAFP

Section 1
Code Algorithms

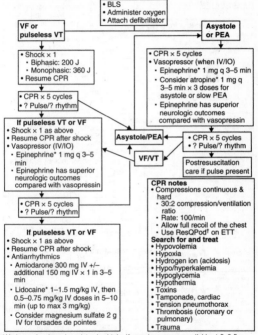

- BLS
- Administer oxygen
- Attach defibrillator

VF or pulseless VT

- Shock × 1
  - Biphasic: 200 J
  - Monophasic: 360 J
  - Resume CPR

- CPR × 5 cycles
- ? Pulse/? rhythm

If pulseless VT or VF
- Shock × 1 as above
- Resume CPR after shock
- Vasopressor (IV/IO)
  - Epinephrine* 1 mg q 3–5 min
  - Epinephrine has superior neurologic outcomes compared with vasopressin

- CPR × 5 cycles
- ? Pulse/? rhythm

If pulseless VT or VF
- Shock × 1 as above
- Resume CPR after shock
- Antiarrhythmics
  - Amiodarone 300 mg IV +/– additional 150 mg IV × 1 in 3–5 min
  - Lidocaine* 1–1.5 mg/kg IV, then 0.5–0.75 mg/kg IV doses in 5–10 min (up to max 3 mg/kg)
  - Consider magnesium sulfate 2 g IV for torsades de pointes

Asystole or PEA

- CPR × 5 cycles
- Vasopressor (when IV/IO)
  - Epinephrine* 1 mg q 3–5 min
  - Consider atropine* 1 mg q 3–5 min × 3 doses for asystole or slow PEA
  - Epinephrine has superior neurologic outcomes compared with vasopressin

Asystole/PEA

VF/VT

- CPR × 5 cycles
- ? Pulse/? rhythm

Postresuscitation care if pulse present

CPR notes
- Compressions continuous & hard
  - 30:2 compression/ventilation ratio
  - Rate: 100/min
  - Allow full recoil of the chest
  - Use ResQPod† on ETT
Search for and treat
- Hypovolemia
- Hypoxia
- Hydrogen ion (acidosis)
- Hypo/hyperkalemia
- Hypoglycemia
- Hypothermia
- Toxins
- Tamponade, cardiac
- Tension pneumothorax
- Thrombosis (coronary or pulmonary)
- Trauma

*Meds may be given via endotracheal tube if vascular access unavailable at 2–2.5 × standard IV doses.

†ResQPOD is an impedance threshold device that increases blood flow to the heart and brain during CPR.

Adapted from 2005 American Heart Association Guidelines for Cardiopulmonary Resuscitation and Emergency Cardiovascular Care. *Circulation* 2005;112(24 suppl) and *NEJM* 2008;359:21.

Figure 1-1 Pulseless Arrest Algorithm

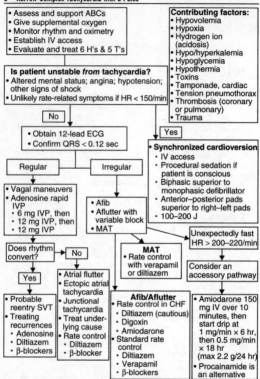

Adapted from 2005 American Heart Association Guidelines for Cardiopulmonary Resuscitation and Emergency Cardiovascular Care. *Circulation* 2005;112(24 suppl).

Figure 1-2 Narrow-Complex Tachycardia with a Pulse

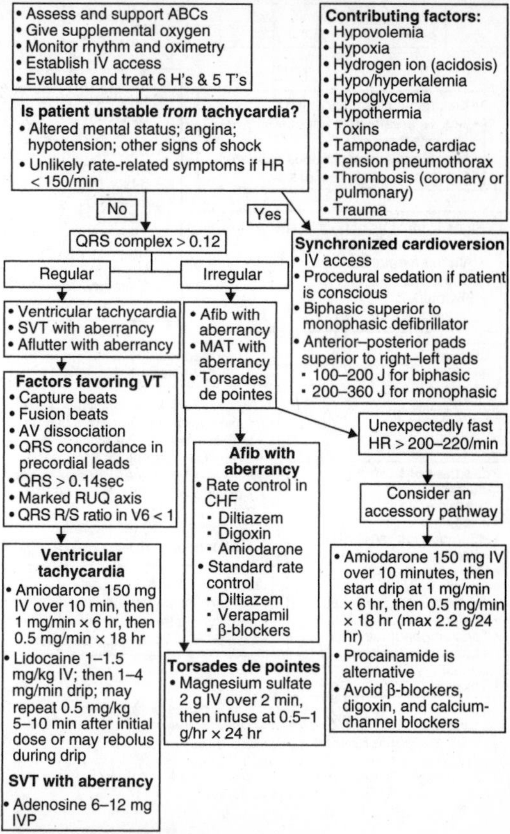

- Assess and support ABCs
- Give supplemental oxygen
- Monitor rhythm and oximetry
- Establish IV access
- Evaluate and treat 6 H's & 5 T's

Contributing factors:
- Hypovolemia
- Hypoxia
- Hydrogen ion (acidosis)
- Hypo/hyperkalemia
- Hypoglycemia
- Hypothermia
- Toxins
- Tamponade, cardiac
- Tension pneumothorax
- Thrombosis (coronary or pulmonary)
- Trauma

Is patient unstable *from* tachycardia?
- Altered mental status; angina; hypotension; other signs of shock
- Unlikely rate-related symptoms if HR < 150/min

No → QRS complex > 0.12

Yes →

Synchronized cardioversion
- IV access
- Procedural sedation if patient is conscious
- Biphasic superior to monophasic defibrillator
- Anterior–posterior pads superior to right–left pads
  - 100–200 J for biphasic
  - 200–360 J for monophasic

QRS complex > 0.12

Regular | Irregular

Regular:
- Ventricular tachycardia
- SVT with aberrancy
- Aflutter with aberrancy

Irregular:
- Afib with aberrancy
- MAT with aberrancy
- Torsades de pointes

Factors favoring VT
- Capture beats
- Fusion beats
- AV dissociation
- QRS concordance in precordial leads
- QRS > 0.14sec
- Marked RUQ axis
- QRS R/S ratio in V6 < 1

Afib with aberrancy
- Rate control in CHF
  - Diltiazem
  - Digoxin
  - Amiodarone
- Standard rate control
  - Diltiazem
  - Verapamil
  - β-blockers

Unexpectedly fast HR > 200–220/min

↓

Consider an accessory pathway

↓

- Amiodarone 150 mg IV over 10 minutes, then start drip at 1 mg/min × 6 hr, then 0.5 mg/min × 18 hr (max 2.2 g/24 hr)
- Procainamide is alternative
- Avoid β-blockers, digoxin, and calcium-channel blockers

Ventricular tachycardia
- Amiodarone 150 mg IV over 10 min, then 1 mg/min × 6 hr, then 0.5 mg/min × 18 hr
- Lidocaine 1–1.5 mg/kg IV; then 1–4 mg/min drip; may repeat 0.5 mg/kg 5–10 min after initial dose or may rebolus during drip

SVT with aberrancy
- Adenosine 6–12 mg IVP

Torsades de pointes
- Magnesium sulfate 2 g IV over 2 min, then infuse at 0.5–1 g/hr × 24 hr

Adapted from *Circulation* 2005;112(Suppl 24).

Figure 1-3 Wide-Complex Tachycardia with a Pulse

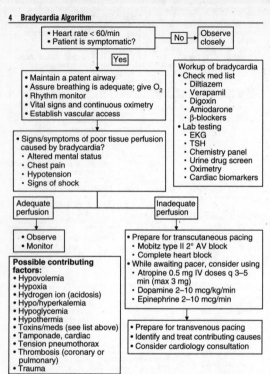

Adapted from 2005 American Heart Association Guidelines for Cardiopulmonary Resuscitation and Emergency Cardiovascular Care. *Circulation* 2005;112(24 suppl).

Figure 1-4 Bradycardia Algorithm

Table 1-1 Basic Life Support for Healthcare Providers

Maneuver	Adolescent and older	One year to adolescent	Infant under 1 year of age
Airway	If no suspected neck trauma: head tilt/chin lift If suspected neck trauma: jaw thrust		
Rescue breathing without chest compressions	1 breath every 5-6 sec	1 breath every 3-5 sec	
Rescue breathing for CPR with advanced airway	1 breath every 6-8 sec		
Airway obstructed by foreign body	Abdominal thrusts		Up to 5 repetitions of back slaps and chest thrusts
Circulation	Check carotid pulse for up to 10 sec		Check brachial or femoral pulses for up to 10 sec
Compression site	Lower sternum between nipples	Sternum just below nipple line	
Compression method: push hard and fast and allow complete recoil; if two providers, no pauses for ventilation	Heel of one hand with other hand on top	Heel of one hand	2 fingers (lone provider) or 2 thumbs and encircling hands (two providers)
Compression depth	1.5-2 inches	1/3 to 1/2 the depth of the chest	
Compression rate	Approximately 100 beats/min		
Compression-ventilation ratio	30:2 (one or two providers)	30:2 (lone provider) 15:2 (two providers)	
Defibrillation AED	Use adult pads	Witnessed collapse or hospital arrest: use AED immediately with pediatric pads (if available)	No recommendation

Adapted from 2005 American Heart Association Guidelines for Cardiopulmonary Resuscitation and Emergency Cardiovascular Care. *Circulation* 2005;112(24 suppl).

Section 2
General Issues in Hospital Medicine

NUTRITIONAL GUIDELINES FOR HOSPITALIZED PATIENTS

- If GI tract is functional, use **enteral** support before resorting to parenteral nutrition. Enteral nutrition (EN) compared to parenteral nutrition (PN) is associated with a significant reduction in the number of infectious complications.
- **Caloric requirement in non-ICU patients** is based on a calculation of the resting energy expenditure (REE in kcal/day) using the Harris-Benedict equation:
  - ➤ Men: REE = 66.5 + (13.75 × wt [kg]) + (5 × ht [cm]) − (6.76 × age [yr])
  - ➤ Women: REE = 655 + (9.56 × wt [kg]) + (1.85 × ht [cm]) − (4.68 × age [yr])
- In hemodynamically stable ICU pts, start EN within 24–48 hr of injury or admission
  - ➤ Early enteral nutrition is associated with a trend toward reduction in mortality and reduction of infectious complications in critically ill patients
  - ➤ Estimate caloric needs in critically ill patients using actual body weights (ABW)
    - ○ 20–25 kcal/kg/day during the **initial** acute phase of critical illness
    - ○ Advance to 25–30 kcal/kg/day during the anabolic or recovery phase of illness
    - ○ Obese (BMI > 30): consider permissive underfeeding at 11–14 kcal/kg/d ABW
    - ○ Avoid overfeeding: leads to hyperglycemia, fatty liver, hypertriglyceridemia, immune suppression, inflammatory response, hypercapnia, and azotemia
- **Estimating protein needs** based on level of stress and level of renal impairment
  - ➤ Normal renal function and low stress: 0.8–1.2 g/kg/d; moderate stress: 1.3–1.5 g/kg/d; high stress or ICU: 1.5–2 g/kg/d (based on ideal weight if obese)
  - ➤ Hemodialysis: low stress = 1–1.4 g/kg/d; high stress or ICU = 2–2.5 g/kg/d
  - ➤ No protein restrictions for hepatic encephalopathy or for CKD without dialysis
- **Indications for specialized enteral formulas**
  - ➤ Immunomodulating formulas (with arginine, glutamine, nucleic acid, omega-3 fatty acids, and antioxidants [e.g., Impact]) indicated after major surgery, severe trauma, burns, head/neck cancer, and critically ill ventilated patients **who are not septic**
  - ➤ Enteral formulas with omega-3 fatty acids, gamma-linolenic acid, and antioxidants (e.g., Oxepa) are indicated for severe sepsis, ARDS, or acute lung injury
- Adjunctive therapy
  - ➤ Unclear benefit of probiotics after major trauma, abdominal surgery, or transplantation
  - ➤ Selenium 400 mcg IV daily may help for burns, trauma, ARDS, or septic shock
- **When to use parenteral nutrition (PN)**
  - ➤ If a patient with malnutrition or a catabolic state is unable to tolerate enteral diet ≥5 d
  - ➤ Consider supplemental PN if far from enteral nutrition goals after 7–10 d
  - ➤ In malnourished patients, consider initiating PN 5–7 d before a major operation and continuing it postop if enteral nutrition will not be tolerated early postop
  - ➤ If malnourished ICU pt cannot tolerate EN, may start PN soon after pt resuscitated
    - ○ Propofol adds lipid and calories (1.1 cal or 0.1 g lipid/mL) and affects PN orders

- **Monitoring nutritional support**
  - No value in following albumin, prealbumin, transferrin, retinol-binding protein, or anthropometry to monitor nutritional support in the ICU
  - Follow weekly weights
  - Nitrogen balance = nitrogen intake (g protein/6.25 or appropriate conversion) minus nitrogen losses (UUN excretion in g + 3–5 g "fudge factor")
    - Feeding should be stable at goal rate for at least 2–3 d prior to collection
    - Desire a positive nitrogen balance to assure an anabolic state
  - Tube feedings—monitor the following for tolerance of gastric tube feeds:
    - Abdominal pain or distention, nausea/vomiting, and stool frequency
    - Avoid holding gastric tube feeds unless residuals >400–500 mL or other signs of tube feeding intolerance are present; keep head of bed elevated >30°
    - Consider metoclopramide or erythromycin for persistent residuals >250 mL
    - NGT drainage of 1.2 L/d is approximate cutoff for initiation of gastric feeds
    - Consider jejunal feeds if: lack of accessible stomach, gastric outlet obstruction, gastric feeding intolerance, or at a high risk for gastric aspiration (gastric feeds or jejunal feeds may be used for severe acute pancreatitis)
- **How to advance tube feedings**
  - Start tube feeding rate at 20–25 mL/hr
  - Advance 10–25 mL every 6–8 hr as tolerated
  - Consider advancing slower if: pt has not been fed for >7 d; risk for refeeding syndrome; has received long-term PN; history of a significant bowel resection; impaired gastric emptying; presence of bowel wall edema, multiple bowel re-explorations, or an open abdominal cavity; receipt of a calorie-dense or high-osmolality formula (e.g., 2CalHN or Nepro); or presence of gut hypoperfusion, hypotension, or hemodynamic instability

References: J Parenteral Enteral Nutr 2009;33:277 and Clinical Nutr 2006;25:210. Adapted with permission from Patty Manpearl, RD.

PAIN MANAGEMENT IN THE HOSPITALIZED PATIENT

Stepwise Approach to Medication Management of Acute Pain
- Mild pain: acetaminophen, NSAIDs, or salicylates (Table 2-1)
- Moderate pain: add low-dose opioids often as combination products (acetaminophen with hydrocodone or codeine), or tramadol (if no history of seizures and no serotonergic drug therapy) (Table 2-4)
  - For mild to moderate pain, meds should be titrated to effect then given on a scheduled basis.
- Moderate to severe pain: give scheduled analgesics with as-needed meds for breakthrough pain
  - Use standardized pain scales and reassess pain with each vital sign check.
  - Rescue dose is 10–15% of 24-hr daily dose q 2–4 hr as needed.
- Severe pain: parenteral opioids (Tables 2-2 and 2-3)
- Neuropathic pain: best managed by adjuvant medications listed in Table 2-4

Patient-Controlled Analgesia (PCA)
- Neither family nor staff may administer opioid doses to patient
- Administered doses: morphine 1–2 mg; hydromorphone 0.1–0.3 mg; fentanyl 10–20 mcg
  - If pain inadequately controlled after 1 hr, ↑ dose 25–50% per dose until pain controlled

Table 2-1 Non-Opioid Analgesics

Medication	Usual oral adult dose	Max daily adult dose	Usual oral pediatric dose
acetaminophen	650 mg q4–6h	4000 mg*	10–15 mg/kg q4–6h
Salicylates[†]			
aspirin	325–650 mg q4–6h	4000 mg	N/R for <19 yr[‡]
diflunisal	500 mg q12h	1500 mg	N/R
salsalate	500 mg q4h	3000 mg	N/R
trilisate	1000–1500 mg q12h	3000 mg	N/R
Nonsteroidal anti-inflammatory drugs (NSAIDs)[§]			
diclofenac	50 mg q8h	150 mg	N/R
flurbiprofen	50–100 mg bid–tid	300 mg	N/R
ibuprofen	400–800 mg q6–8h	3200 mg	10 mg/kg q6–8h
indomethacin	25–50 mg q8h	200 mg	0.3–1 mg/kg q6–8h
ketoprofen	25–75 mg q6–8h	300 mg	N/R
ketorolac[¶]	10 mg PO q6–8h 30 mg IV/IM q6h (<65 yr) 15 mg IV/IM q6h (>65 yr)	120 mg (<65 yr) 60 mg (>65 yr)	0.5 mg/kg PO/IV/IM q6h (max 100 mg/day)
meclofenamate	50–100 mg q4–6h	400 mg	N/R
mefenamic acid	250 mg q6h[‖]	1250 mg × 1 then 1 g/d	N/R
nabumetone	500–1000 mg bid	2000 mg	N/R
naproxen	250–500 mg bid	1000 mg	5–10 mg/kg q12h
naproxen sodium	275–550 mg bid	1100 mg	5–10 mg/kg q12h
oxaprozin	1200 mg daily	1800 mg	10–20 mg/kg daily
piroxicam	20 mg daily	20 mg	N/R
sulindac	150–200 mg q12h	400 mg	N/R
tolmetin	200–600 mg tid	1800 mg	N/R
Medications with significant cyclooxygenase-2-selective (COX-2) inhibition[#]			
celecoxib[¶]	100–200 mg bid	400 mg	N/R
etodolac	200–400 mg q6–8h	1200 mg	N/R
meloxicam	7.5 mg daily	15 mg	N/R

*Maximum dose of acetaminophen is 2 g/d if the patient is an alcoholic, is severely malnourished, or has advanced cirrhosis.
† Salicylates as a class are associated with increased risk of gastritis or peptic ulcer disease, reversible inhibition of platelet aggregation (except aspirin is irreversible), potential papillary necrosis of kidneys, and possible exacerbation of asthma.
‡ Salicylate use during a viral illness in patient ≤18 years may cause Reye's syndrome.
§ NSAIDs as a class are associated with increased risk of gastritis or peptic ulcer disease, reversible inhibition of platelet aggregation, potential papillary necrosis of kidneys, and possible fluid retention and elevated blood pressure; ibuprofen can offset the antiplatelet action of aspirin.
‖ Duration of use limited to 5 days. Ketorolac only NSAID available in a parenteral formulation.
¶ Brand name medications only (not available as low-cost generics, as is true of the others in this table).
# These agents have the same GI toxicity as nonselective NSAIDs, have little effect on platelet aggregation, and can cause papillary necrosis of the kidneys. Rofecoxib (Vioxx) and valdecoxib (Bextra) were withdrawn from the market for their association with an increased risk of MI and stroke.
Adapted from the Principles of Analgesic Use in the Treatment of Acute Pain and Cancer Pain, 5th Edition. American Pain Society, 2003, and *Am Fam Phys* 2005;71:913–918.

Table 2-2 Fentanyl Transdermal Dose (based on ongoing morphine requirement)*†

Morphine (IV/IM)	Morphine (PO)	Transdermal Fentanyl
10–22 mg/day	60–134 mg/day	25 mcg/hr
23–37 mg/day	135–224 mg/day	50 mcg/hr
38–52 mg/day	225–314 mg/day	75 mcg/hr
53–67 mg/day	315–404 mg/day	100 mcg/hr

* For higher morphine doses, see product insert for transdermal fentanyl equivalencies.
† Anticipate a delay in 12–18 hr for full analgesic effect of transdermal fentanyl.
Not for use in acute pain management, for opiate-naïve pts, or for pain that is not constant.
Adapted from Ortho-McNeil package insert at www.duragesic.com.

Table 2-3 Opioid Equivalency*

Opioid	PO	IV/SC/IM	Opioid	PO	IV/SC/IM
buprenorphine	n/a	0.3–0.4 mg	meperidine†	300 mg	100 mg
butorphanol	n/a	2 mg	methadone	5–15 mg	2.5–10 mg
codeine	130 mg	75 mg	morphine	30 mg	10 mg
fentanyl	n/a	0.1 mg	nalbuphine	n/a	20 mg
hydrocodone	30 mg	n/a	oxycodone	20 mg	n/a
hydromorphone	7.5 mg	1.5 mg	oxymorphone	10 mg	1 mg
levorphanol	4 mg	2 mg	pentazocine	150 mg	60 mg

* Approximate equianalgesic doses as adapted from the 2003 and 2005 American Pain Society (www.ampainsoc.org) guidelines and the 1992 AHCPR guidelines.
† Doses should be limited to <600 mg/24 hr and total duration of use <48 hr; meperidine should **not** be used for chronic pain management.
n/a = Not available. See drug entries themselves for starting doses. Recommend using 25% lower than equivalent doses when switching between opioids. IV doses should be titrated slowly with appropriate monitoring. All PO dosing is with immediate-release preparations. Individualize all dosing, especially in the elderly, in children, and in those who are opioid naïve, have chronic pain, or have hepatic/renal insufficiency. Adapted with permission from the *Tarascon Pocket Pharmacopoeia*, 2009.

- Lockout interval: typically 10 min
- Basal rate: none for opioid-naïve pts; use equianalgesic infusion for pts on chronic opioids
  - ➤ May increase basal rate up to 50% q 8 hr if needed to optimize pain control

Management of Opioid Side Effects
- Constipation: scheduled prophylactic docusate and a stimulant agent (e.g., Peri-Colace or Senna Plus); tolerance does not develop
- Sedation: tolerance develops in 48–72 hr; may reduce dose and hold other sedatives
- Nausea/vomiting: tolerance develops in 48–72 hr; may reduce dose, change opioid, or give a trial of antiemetic (e.g., metoclopramide) if symptoms are intolerable
- Pruritus: dose reduction, change opioid, or 2nd-generation antihistamine (e.g., loratadine)
- Hallucinations/confusion: dose reduction; change opioid; trial of haloperidol or risperidone
- Respiratory depression: hold opioid; naloxone 0.1 mg IV q 30–60 sec titrated to effect

Adjuvant Treatments for Inflammatory Pain Syndromes
- Epidural steroid injections for cervical or lumbar radiculopathy

Table 2-4 Adjuvant Medications for Neuropathic Pain

Medication	Starting oral adult dose	Titration/Usual oral daily dose range in mg	Numbers needed to treat (NNT$_{50}$) *
Antiepileptics			
carbamazepine	100 mg bid	100 mg q7d / 1000–1600†	2.6–3.3
clonazepam‡	0.5 mg daily	0.5 mg q3–5d / 5–20	—
gabapentin§	100–300 mg qhs	300 mg q7d / 1800–3600	3.2–4.1
lamotrigine	25–50 mg daily	25 mg q7d / 200–600	2.1
phenytoin	100 mg qhs	100 mg q7d / 300	—
pregabalin‖	50 mg tid	150 mg q7d / 300–600	—
topiramate	25 mg daily	25 mg q7d / 400–800	—
Tricyclic antidepressants			
amitriptyline	10 mg qhs	10 mg q7d / 50–150†	1.3–3.0
desipramine	25 mg qhs	25 mg q7d / 75–200†	1.3–3.0
doxepin	10 mg qhs	10 mg q7d / 75–150	1.3–3.0
nortriptyline	10 mg qhs	10 mg q7d / 25–75†	1.3–3.0
Selective serotonin reuptake inhibitors (SSRIs)‡			
paroxetine	10 mg daily	10 mg q7d / 20–60	6.7
citalopram	10 mg daily	10 mg q7d / 20–60	6.7
Other antidepressants			
duloxetine‖	30 mg daily	30 mg q14d / 30–120	—
milnacipran‖	12.5 mg daily	12.5–25 mg q7d / 100–200	—
venlafaxine	37.5 mg daily	37.5 mg q7d / 150–300	—
Topical anesthetic creams			
capsaicin	0.25% tid	Use up to 0.75% 5 times/d	5.3–5.9
5% lidoderm‖	1 patch bid	Use up to 3 patches bid	4.4
Miscellaneous analgesics			
dextromethorphan	30 mg bid	30 mg q7d / 60 mg q6h	1.9‡
tramadol	50 mg bid	50 mg q7d / 400	3.1–3.4
Opioid analgesics (as extended-release or controlled-release formulations)			
morphine SR	15 mg bid	15 mg q7d / 60–360	—
oxycodone SR‖	10 mg bid	10 mg q7d / 20–160	2.5
methadone	2.5 mg bid	2.5 mg q7d until qid / 10–80	—

* NNT$_{50}$ is the number needed to treat to decrease the neuropathic pain severity ≥50% in one patient.
† Titrate drug dosage to therapeutic effect; serum drug levels available to guide dosing.
‡ Data supporting the efficacy of SSRIs, benzodiazepines, and dextromethorphan for neuropathic or functional pain syndromes is sparse.
§ Gabapentin + sustained-release morphine more effective than either agent alone (*NEJM* 2005;352:1324).
‖ Brand name medication only (not available as a low-cost generic, as is true of the other meds in this table).
Adapted from: *NEJM* 2003;348:1243; *NEJM* 2003;349:1943; *Mayo Clin Proc* 2004;79:1533; *Pain* 2003;106:151; *Curr Opin Anaesth* 2006;19:573; *Mayo Clin Proc* 2006;81:S3; *J Fam Prac* 2007;56:3; and the Pain Management Guidelines of the Institute for Clinical Systems Improvement at www.icsi.org.

- Pain from bone metastases: radiation therapy +/− dexamethasone 4–8 mg PO q 8–12 hr
  - ➤ Strontium or samarium are alternative treatments for painful bone metastases.
- Vertebral compression fractures: calcitonin 200 units intranasally daily and use a TLSO brace
- Muscle spasticity: start baclofen 5–10 mg PO tid–qid (titrate to max of 80 mg/day)

Epidural Analgesia
- Consider for postop analgesia after major abdominal, thoracic, orthopedic, or gyn operations
- Avoid antithrombotics/anticoagulants for 24 hr prior to discontinuation of epidural catheters

References: Mayo Clin Proc *2004;79:1533;* NEJM *2003;348:1243 and 349:1943;* Ann Int Med *2004;140:441;* Cancer J *2006;12:330;* J Palliative Med *2006;9:1414;* J Am Coll Surg *2006;202:169;* 2004 guidelines at www.icsi.org.

ETHICAL ISSUES IN THE HOSPITAL

Core Ethical Principles
- Advance directives act as a guide for the patient's wishes at the end of life and must be followed.
- Patients have autonomy and the right to self-determination for all medical decisions.
  - ➤ Adults with decision-making capacity have the right to refuse/accept any interventions.
  - ➤ A patient or his/her surrogate does **not** have the right to demand a particular intervention.
- For patients incapable of making a decision, a surrogate decision maker must make a decision on behalf of the patient in a way that is **consistent with the patient's set of values**.
- If the patient's wishes are not known by the family and there is no durable power of attorney, the family is obligated to make decisions based on the **presumed wishes of the patient** (i.e., substituted judgment).
- Physicians should treat all patients with respect, beneficence, justice, and nonmaleficence.
- Despite contrary wishes, a physician is not obligated to continue any futile medical care.

Resolving Conflict
- Need to understand the patient's goals of treatment (cure, prolonging life, or palliation)
- Arbitration if the patient/family insists on an intervention that the clinician(s) feel is inadvisable
  - ➤ Hospital ethics committees are ideally suited to resolve conflicts over end-of-life issues.

References: Crit Care Med *2007;35:S85;* Crit Care Med *2008;36:953.*

PALLIATIVE AND END-OF-LIFE CARE IN THE HOSPITAL

Six Steps to Breaking Bad News
1. Meet with the patient and any close family members to review the medical history.
2. Find out how much the patient knows about his/her diagnosis and prognosis.

3. Determine how much the patient wants to know and who else may know.
4. Share the bad news succinctly and using simple language. Allow time for patient to absorb and react to the news. Ask the patient to repeat what was said.
5. Respond to the patient's feelings. Acknowledge emotions and provide support.
6. Create a plan of care, and assure patient that you will not abandon him/her.

VALUE Mnemonic for Family Conferences
- **V**alue the statements made by family members.
- **A**cknowledge the emotions of family members (have tissues available).
- **L**isten carefully to the various family members.
- **U**nderstand who the patient is as a person (his/her values and expressed wishes).
- **E**licit questions from family members about their concerns, and have **E**mpathy.

Table 2-5 Common Distressing Symptoms Amenable to Palliation

Symptom	Potential therapies
Anxiety/agitation	Lorazepam 0.5–2 mg or alprazolam 0.25–1 mg PO q2–4h prn
Dyspnea	Oxygen (if hypoxic); fan; bronchodilators; morphine (if severe)
Anorexia	Mirtazapine; megestrol; prednisone or dronabinol
Delirium	Haloperidol 0.5–1 mg PO/SL/IM bid–tid; verbal reorientation; zolendronate 4 mg IV or pamidronate 60 mg IV if due to ↑↑ Ca^{2+}
Constipation	Docusate and senna or lactulose
Coughing	Acetaminophen with codeine elixir or benzonatate tabs prn
Depression	SSRI; mirtazapine (if anorexia present)
Diarrhea	Soluble fiber; loperamide or diphenoxylate and atropine prn
Dysphagia	Thickened liquids; pureed foods; consider feeding tube if severe
Edema	Loop diuretics; elevate extremities
Fatigue	Treat depression if present; methylphenidate 2.5–5 mg PO q AM
Fever	Acetaminophen; NSAIDs; fan; cool wash cloths
Hiccuping	Thorazine 25–50 mg PO/IM tid–qid prn
Nausea	Prochlorperazine; metoclopramide; ondansetron; dronabinol prn; lorazepam; dexamethasone 4–8 mg PO bid; or olanzapine
Pain	Mild—aspirin, acetaminophen, or NSAIDs Moderate—acetaminophen/opioid products or tramadol Severe—Opioids (morphine, hydromorphone, methadone, levorphanol, fentanyl, or oxycodone) • Use **scheduled oral** formulations if possible • Increase daily opioid dose 25% for mild pain, 25–50% for moderate pain, and 100% for severe pain • Short-acting opioid at 10–15% daily dose q1h as needed for breakthrough pain
Muscle spasms	Clonazepam 0.5 mg PO bid; baclofen 5–10 mg PO tid; +/– opioid
Pruritus	Hydration, emollients, switch opioids, and antihistamines prn
Excessive secretions	Scopolamine 1.5-mg patch behind ear q72h; or atropine 1% solution, 2–3 gtts sublingual q1–2h prn
Xerostomia	Glycerin swabs; lemon drops; vaseline ointment to lips

Adapted from *Amer Fam Physician* 2008;77:167–174.

End-of-Life Decision Making
- Encourage patients to complete a written advance directive for health care.
- Ascertain what the patient's goals of care are for health at the end of life.
  - ➢ What are the patient's fears and hopes regarding the end of life?
- An advance directive should include preferences about cardiopulmonary resuscitation, defibrillation, intubation, dialysis, vasopressor use, transfusion of blood products, antibiotic use, and artificial hydration/nutrition (i.e., feeding tubes).

Withholding Versus Withdrawing Care
- Legally and philosophically there is no distinction between these 2 actions

Allow Natural Death (AND)
- AND begins once the decision has been made to focus efforts on patient comfort.
- Terminal sedation and euthanasia are very different because of differences in intent.
  - ➢ Terminal sedation utilizes opioids and anxiolytics with the intent to prevent pain, anxiety, or dyspnea; euthanasia uses medicines with the intent to cause death
  - ➢ Symptoms controlled with a morphine infusion and intermittent IV lorazepam
  - ➢ Haloperidol 5 mg IV q1h prn for agitated delirium
- Spiritual considerations: Ask the family if they want a religious representative to visit.

Organ Donation
- The organ procurement agency affiliated with the hospital should be contacted once the decision has been made to withdraw life-sustaining support. This agency, not the treating physicians, should approach the family to discuss organ donation.

Eligibility Guidelines for Hospice
- Terminal illness with life expectancy of 6 months or less
- Patient elects treatment goals directed toward symptom relief versus disease cure
- Patient has had a marked functional decline and/or critical nutritional impairment
- Disease-specific criteria for end-stage disease: incurable cancer, severe dementia, end-stage heart or lung disease, end-stage AIDS, neurologic disease with critically impaired breathing or incapacity to eat, end-stage kidney disease not seeking dialysis, any terminal illness with a rapid decline, inability to eat, hypotension, or requires assistance with most activities of daily living

Adapted from Clinical Practice Guidelines for Quality Palliative Care, 2004. *Available at www.nationalconsensusproject.org/Guideline.pdf.* Amer Fam Physician *2008;77:167–174.*

Section 3
Basics of Hospital Care of the Geriatric Patient

FUNCTIONAL ASSESSMENT OF ELDERLY PATIENTS

Table 3-1 Activities of Daily Living and Instrumental Activities of Daily Living

Independence with ADLs (DEATH)	Independence with IADLs (SHAFT)
D—Dressing	S—Shopping
E—Eating	H—Housework
A—Ambulating and ability to transfer	A—Accounting
T—Toileting and continence	F—Food preparation
H—Hygiene (bathing)	T—Transportation and use of telephone

Table 3-2 Get Up and Go Test for Geriatric Mobility

	Seconds	Rating
Get up and go predictive results	<10	Freely mobile
	10–19	Fairly independent
	≥20	Impaired mobility

Test: Get up out of a standard armchair, walk 3 m (10 ft), turn, walk back to chair and sit down. Ambulate with or without an assistive device and follow the table's 3-step command. One practice trial and 3 actual trials are performed, with the 3 trials averaged.
Adapted from *J Am Geriatric Soc* 1991;39:142–148.

Assessment for Protein-Calorie Malnutrition
- Exam: low body weight, recent weight loss, pressure sores, brittle hair and nails, sunken eyes, pale sclera, little subcutaneous fat, temporal muscle wasting, and muscle atrophy
- Labs: serum albumin < 3.5 g/dL; prealbumin < 15 mg/dL; transferrin < 200 mg/dL; and total lymphocyte count < 1500/mm^3
- Risk factors for malnutrition: poor dentition, dry mouth, poverty, inability to obtain or prepare food, comorbid medical conditions, malabsorption, altered taste, and mood disorders

Vision Screen
- Includes a visual acuity screen and fundoscopic exam
- Impaired vision from cataracts, macular degeneration, glaucoma, or refractive error

Hearing Screen
- Includes check for ability to hear a whispered voice and an otoscopic exam
- Impaired hearing from presbycusis, cerumen impaction, otosclerosis, or acoustic neuroma

Rapid Depression Screen for Elderly Patients
Inquire about the following 3 areas:
- "Have you been feeling sad or depressed?"; any anhedonia; any sleep disturbances
- Use the 15-item Geriatric Depression Scale if any of these items are present

Cognitive Assessment in the Elderly

- Mini-cog screen for cognitive impairment: 3-item immediate recall; clock draw test (ask patient to draw a clock and place the hands to read "10 after 11"); 3-item delayed recall
- Folstein mini-mental status exam if the mini-cog screen is abnormal (Table 3-3)

Table 3-3 Folstein Mini-Mental Status Exam

Cognitive Screening Test

Part I: Direct Patient Testing

1. Information for Delayed Recall Test
   A. Give the patient a name and address to remember and recite it. Tell them to remember this information because you will ask about it again in a few minutes.
   B. Patient may make 4 attempts to correctly recite the information
   C. Example: Joe Smith, 54 Circle Drive, Dallas
   D. No points given for immediate recall

2. Time Orientation Test
   A. Ask the patient, "What is the date?"
   B. Patient must give the month, day, and year
   C. 1 point for an exact answer

3. Clock Drawing Test
   A. Give the patient a blank piece of paper
   B. Ask them to draw a clock face including all the numbers to indicate the hours of a clock
   C. Then, draw the hands of the clock to show a time of eleven fifteen (11:15)
   D. Two points possible: one point for part B and one point for part C

4. Recent Events Test
   A. Have the patient tell you something that has happened in the news recently (either national or local news item is acceptable)
   B. Patient must give a specific answer
   C. 1 point for a specific correct answer

5. Delayed Recall Test
   A. Ask the patient to recite the name and address they were asked to remember
   B. 5 points possible: 1 point each for first name, last name, street number, street name, and city

Scoring
A. A score of 9 signifies no significant impairment in cognition
B. Score of 5–8 if indeterminate; further testing is required
C. Score of 4 or below signifies cognitive impairment; further detailed testing is required to assess the degree of cognitive impairment

Part II: Family/Acquaintance Interview

Ask the friend or family member of the patient the following questions:
1. Does (name of patient) have more trouble remembering recent events now compared with before?
2. Does (name of patient) have more trouble remembering recent conversations a few days after they have happened*?
3. Has (name of patient) had more trouble finding the right word to say or use wrong words while speaking?
4. Is (name of patient) less capable of managing his/her finances recently†?
5. Is (name of patient) less capable of managing his/her medications recently‡?
6. Does (name of patient) need more help with transportation to and from places†?

* Trouble remembering is due to cognitive impairment and not hearing impairment
† Trouble is due to cognitive impairment and not visual impairment
‡ Trouble is due to cognitive impairment and not physical impairment requiring assistance

Scoring
A. Each question can be answered "yes," "no," "don't know," or "not applicable"
B. Give 1 point to all answers that are either "no," "don't know," or "not applicable"
C. A total score of 0–3 indicates that cognitive impairment is present and that further detailed testing is indicated

Source: Adapted from *J Amer Geriatric Society*; 2002; Vol 50 (Issue 3): 530–34.

PRESSURE ULCERS

- **Risk factors:** malnutrition, immobility, dry skin, low body weight, multiple medical comorbidities, immunosuppression, coma, excessive local moisture, and lymphopenia (Table 3-4)
- **Indications for antibiotics:** presence of cellulitis, osteomyelitis, or systemic infection

INTERVENTIONS TO PREVENT NOSOCOMIAL COMPLICATIONS IN THE HOSPITAL

- **Preventing Functional Decline**
  - ➤ Early mobility with physical and occupational therapy: limit bed rest
  - ➤ Assess the need for an assistive device to be used for ambulation
  - ➤ Aggressive nutritional support under the guidance of a certified dietician

Table 3-4 Staging and Treatment of Pressure Ulcers

Stage	Description	Treatment
I	Nonblanchable erythema of intact skin	Turn pt side-to-side to an oblique angle q2h; keep head of bed ≤30°
II	Skin loss involving epidermis +/– dermis	Above; nonocclusive moist dressing; pressure-reducing devices*
III	Full thickness skin loss to subcutaneous tissue up to the level of the fascia	Above; debridement; hydrogel, alginate, hydrocolloid or moistened gauze dressings
IV	Full thickness skin loss through fascia	Above; debridement; and surgical repair

HOB = head of bed.
* Static devices: foam, air mattress, or mattress overlays; benefit of dynamic devices is unclear.
Adapted from *Am Fam Physician* 2008;78:1186.

Table 3-5 Evaluation of Elderly Patients Presenting After a Fall

Functional History Concerning a Fall		Key Physical Exam Findings	
C	Caregiver and housing adequate	I	Inflamed joints (or immobility)
A	Alcohol (and withdrawal)	H	Hypotension or orthostasis
T	Treatment (meds, compliance)	A	Auditory or visual abnormalities
A	Affect (depression)	T	Tremor
S	Syncope	E	Equilibrium (disequilibrium)
T	Teetering (dizziness or vertigo)	F	Foot problems
R	Recent medical or surgical illness	A	Arrhythmia, heart block, or valve problem
O	Ocular problems	L	Leg-length discrepancy
P	Pain or problems with mobility	L	Lack of conditioning
H	Hearing impairment	I	Illness—general/medical
E	Environmental hazards (e.g., stairs)	N	Nutrition (weight loss?)
		G	Gait disturbance

Adapted from *Am Fam Physician* 2000;61:2159.

- **Preventing Nosocomial Infections and Inpatient Falls**
  - ➢ Eliminate all unnecessary lines, tubes, and restraints that can impair mobility (Table 3-5)
  - ➢ Avoid bedrails and use of medications listed in Table 3-6
- **Thromboprophylaxis to Prevent Venous Thromboembolism**
  - ➢ Use a low molecular weight heparin (LMWH), or fondaparinux unless contraindicated
    - ○ ↓ dose of LMWH if CrCl 15–30 mL/min; avoid fondaparinux if CrCl < 30 mL/min
  - ➢ Unfractionated heparin 5000 units SQ q8h preferred for CrCl < 15 mL/min
  - ➢ Sequential compression stockings an alternative if thromboprophylaxis contraindicated

Table 3-6 Medications to Use with Extreme Caution in Elderly Patients

alpha-blockers	clonidine	hydroxyzine	oxybutynin
amitriptyline	cyclobenzaprine	hyocyamine	pentazocine
amphetamines	cyproheptadine	indomethacin	perphenazine
barbiturates	dexchlorpheniramine	ketorolac	phenytoin
belladonna alkaloids	diazepam	meperidine	piroxicam
carisoprodol	dicyclomine	meprobamate	promethazine
chlordiazepoxide	diphenhydramine	mesoridazine	propantheline
chlorpheniramine	doxepin	metaxalone	propoxyphene
chlorpropamide	estrogens (high-dose)	methocarbamol	thioridazine
chlorzoxazone	fluoxetine	naproxen	tolterodine
cimetidine	flurazepam	nifedipine (short-acting)	trimethobenzamide
clidinium	glyburide	orphenadrine	zaleplon

Adapted from *Amer J Med* 2007;120:493 and *Arch Int Med* 2003;163:2719.

- **Interventions That Can Minimize the Development of Delirium**
  - ➢ **Risk factors for delirium in the hospital**: dementia; age >65 yr; fracture, infection, or use of antipsychotics or opioids on admission; dehydration; hearing or vision impairment; multiple medical comorbidities; alcohol or drug withdrawal; hypoxia; uncontrolled pain; electrolyte abnormalities; immobility; postop state; and sleep deprivation
  - ➢ **Interventions**: treat underlying cause; constant reorientation with calendars, clocks, dates, lists; early mobility; encourage sitting and full light exposure during daytime to promote wakefulness; visual and hearing aids; attention to fluids to avoid dehydration; avoid hypoxia and electrolyte imbalances; maintain a quiet, dark environment with minimal stimulation at night to enhance sleep; fill room with familiar objects from home; and advise family members and friends to rotate at bedside
  - ➢ **Treatment of delirium**: eliminate all nonessential meds; oral haloperidol 0.5–1 mg bid and q4h prn, risperidone 0.5 mg bid, olanzapine 2.5–5 mg daily, or quetiapine 25 mg bid

References: Am Fam Physician 2008;78:1265; 2008;78:1186; and Gershman K. *The Little Black Book of Geriatrics. 3rd ed. Sudbury, MA: Jones and Bartlett; 2006.*

Section 4
Cardiology

Table 4-1 Life-Threatening Causes of Chest Pain

Condition	Quality	Radiation	Associated signs/symptoms	Exacerbating factors	Relieving factors	Diagnostic studies	Therapy
Acute MI or acute coronary syndrome	Chest pressure heaviness, tightness, Poorly localized	Neck Jaw Shoulders Arms	Nausea Diaphoresis Dyspnea Levine sign	Exertion Emotional distress	Rest Nitrate β-blockers Calcium channel blockers	ECG Cardiac biomarkers Myocardial perfusion studies	See pages 19–21
Pulmonary embolus	Sudden onset Pleuritic chest pain	—	Dyspnea Cough +/– hemoptysis +/– effusion	Deep breaths	Oxygen	CTPA V/Q scan	Heparin or LMWH; TPA for a massive PE
Acute aortic dissection	Sudden onset "tearing" anterior chest pain or back pain	Interscapular area	Δ SBP > 20 mmHg between arms New AI murmur CXR with widened mediastinum	Hypertension Exertion	Rest Blood pressure control	CT angiogram of aortic arch	β-blockers to keep SBP ≤ 110 mmHg and HR < 60 CT surgery consultation
Tension pneumothorax	Sudden onset Unilateral pleuritic chest pain	—	Dyspnea	Exertion Deep breaths	Oxygen Rest	CXR Chest ultrasound	Needle decompression then tube thoracostomy

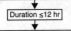

- History of anginal-type CP or anginal equivalent
- ECG, CXR, CHEM-7, CBC, PT, PTT, troponin I
- Establish IV and give oxygen

ECG with ST elevation ≥1 mm in ≥2 contiguous leads **or** new LBBB

Duration ≤12 hr

- Primary PCI + medical rx if door-balloon time or transfer-balloon time within 90 min
  OR
- TPA + Med rx if transfer or door-balloon times not achievable

Primary PCI preferred over TPA
- Cardiogenic shock
  - Adjunctive IABP
- NYHA class III–IV CHF
- Unstable ventricular arrhythmias
- Rescue PCI if < 50% ST-segment resolution by 90 min s/p TPA
- Any contraindication for TPA

Contraindications for TPA
- **Absolute**
  - Prior ICH
  - Brain tumor, aneurysm, AVM
  - Ischemic stroke or closed head injury within 3 months
  - Active internal bleeding
  - Suspected aortic dissection
- **Relative**
  - BP >180/110 mmHg
  - Ischemic stroke > 3 months prior
  - CPR > 10 min
  - Trauma/major surgery w/i 3 wk
  - Internal bleed 2–4 wk ago
  - Noncompressible vessel puncture
  - Pregnancy
  - Current anticoagulation

Duration >12 hr

- Medical therapy
  OR
- Primary PCI + Medical rx for ongoing or recurrent chest pain

Medical therapy for STEMI
- ASA 325 mg chewed, then 162 mg PO daily
- Metoprolol 5 mg IVP q 5 min × 3, then 25–50 mg PO q6h (desire HR 55–65)
- Atorvastatin 80 mg PO daily
- Anticoagulation (choose one of following to be given for entire hospitalization, up to 8 d):
  - Enoxaparin 30 mg IV bolus (< 75 yr) then 1 mg/kg SQ bid
    - 1 mg/kg SQ daily (CrCl 15–30 mL/min)
    - Avoid if CrCl < 15 mL/min
  - Heparin 60 U/kg (max 4,000 units) IV bolus then 12 U/kg/hr (max 1,000 units/hr)
  - Fondaparinux 2.5 mg IV, then 2.5 mg SQ daily; avoid if CrCl < 30 mL/min
- Clopidogrel 300 mg PO × 1, then 75 mg PO daily (usually started after coronary anatomy is known); avoid PPIs
- Nitroglycerin (SL, transdermal, or IV) for persistent chest pain
- Morphine 2 mg IV q 5 min prn severe CP
- GP IIb/IIIa inhibitor added in cath lab
- ACEI started on hospital day 2 as BP allows
  - Earlier if needed for BP control
  - ARB if patient is ACEI-intolerant
- Insulin titrated to chemsticks 80–150 × 48 hr
- Consider eplerenone 25–50 mg PO daily if LVEF ≤0.4 post-MI **and either** DM or CHF

Adapted from: *JACC* 208;51:210; *NEJM* 2007;356:47; *JAMA* 2000;283:2686; and *NEJM* 2006;354:1461.

Figure 4-1 ST-Elevation Myocardial Infarction

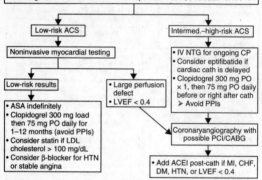

Adapted from: *JACC* 2007;50:654; *Ann Emer Med* 2008;51:591; and *NEJM* 2004;350:1495.

Figure 4-2 Non-ST Elevation Acute Coronary Syndrome

Table 4-2 TIMI Risk Score for Unstable Angina/NSTEMI

TIMI risk score	0–1	2	3	4	5	6–7
Death/MI or urgent revascularization	4.7%	8.3%	13.2%	19.9%	26.2%	40.9%

One point for each variable: age ≥65; ≥3 CAD risk factors; known coronary stenosis ≥50%; ST depressions ≥0.5 mm; ≥2 anginal events within 24 hr; ASA use within 7 d; elevated TnI or CK-MB.
Adapted from *JAMA* 2000;284:835–842.

Table 4-3 Risk of Death or MI in Non-ST Elevation Acute Coronary Syndrome

Characteristics	High-risk ACS (Any of following)	Intermediate-risk ACS (No high-risk; ≥1 of following)	Low-risk ACS (No interm.–high-risk)
History	• Accelerated tempo of ACS sxs ≤ 48 hr	• Prior MI, PVD, CVD, CABG, or ASA use • Age > 70 yr	• Age < 70 yr
Pain	• Ongoing rest angina for at least 20 min	• Rest angina ≥20 min resolved with rest/NTG • Nocturnal angina • Severe/progressive angina ≤ 2 wk	• Increased frequency, severity, or duration of angina • New-onset angina
Exam	• CHF, S_3 or ↑ rales • New/↑ MR murmur • Hypotension • Age >75 yr	—	
ECG	• Rest angina with ST↓ ≥ 0.5 mm • New LBBB • Sustained VT	• Old pathologic Q waves • Diffuse ST↓ <1 mm • T-wave inversions	• Normal ECG or unchanged from baseline
Cardiac enzymes	• TnI ≥ 0.1 ng/mL • ↑ CK-MB	• TnI < 0.1 ng/mL • Slight ↑ CK-MB	• Normal after 6 hr of observation

PVD = peripheral vascular disease; CVD = cerebrovascular disease; MR = mitral regurgitation; NTG = nitroglycerin; ASA = aspirin; LBBB = left bundle branch block; VT = ventricular tachycardia.
Adapted from 2007 ACC/AHA Guideline Update for UA/NSTEMI in *JACC* 2007;50:652–726.

Table 4-4 When Invasive Strategy Preferred Over Conservative Strategy for ACS

• Refractory angina
• TIMI risk score ≥3
• High-risk acute coronary syndrome
• Intermediate-risk NSTEMI
• CHF
• Sustained ventricular tachycardia
• Percutaneous coronary intervention (PCI) in last 6 months
• Prior coronary artery bypass graft (CABG)
• Left ventricular ejection fraction (LVEF) < 0.4
• New ST-segment depressions ≥ 0.5 mm
• High-risk findings on stress test

Adapted from 2007 ACC/AHA Guideline Update for UA/NSTEMI in *JACC* 2007;50:652–726.

Table 4-5 Pretest Probability of Significant CAD with Different Types of Chest Pain

Age (yr)	Nonanginal CP (≤1 of 3 sxs)		Atypical CP (2 of 3 sxs)		Typical CP (3 of 3 sxs)	
	Men	Women	Men	Women	Men	Women
30–39	5%	1%	22%	4%	70%	26%
40–49	14%	3%	46%	13%	87%	55%
50–59	22%	8%	59%	32%	92%	80%
60–69	28%	19%	67%	54%	94%	91%

Symptoms (sxs): substernal CP; CP exacerbated by exertion; CP relieved by NTG or rest.
Adapted from *NEJM* 1979;300:1350.

Table 4-6 Noninvasive Cardiac Testing to Assess for Significant CAD

Test	Indications	Sensitivity	Specificity
Treadmill test*	• Evaluation of CP in low-risk patients • Exercise prescription • Risk stratification post-MI/PCI/CABG • Normal baseline ECG	60–68%	75%
Exercise radionuclide†	• Evaluation of CP in intermediate-risk patients • Abnormal baseline ECG • Better to evaluate atypical CP in women	87%	73%
Adenosine/persantine radionuclide†‡	• Evaluation of CP if unable to exercise • Contraindications: asthma or 2°/3° AV block	89%	75%
Dobutamine radionuclide†	• Evaluation of CP if unable to exercise and adenosine/persantine contraindicated	86%	80–90%
Stress echo	• Evaluation of CP in intermediate-risk patients (operator dependent)	76–92%	75–88%

* Hold β-blockers on morning of exam and hold digoxin ≥ 7 days (if possible).
† Thallium-201 SPECT if pt weight < 250 lbs; ⁹⁹ᵐTc-sestamibi SPECT preferred if weight 250–400 lbs.
‡ No caffeine or theophylline prior to exam.
Adapted from 2003 ACC/AHA Guidelines on Cardiac Radionuclide Imaging available at www.acc.org.

Table 4-7 Non-Life Threatening Causes of Chest Pain

Categories	Pericarditis	Esophageal spasm	GERD (reflux esophagitis)	Costochondritis	Pneumonia (pleurisy)	Zoster	Peptic Ulcers	Acute cholecystitis	Panic attack
Quality	Sharp pain +/- pleuritic	Sharp sub-sternal	Burning	Localized sharp	Pleuritic chest pain	Unilateral burning	Dull pain	Sharp right lower chest	Chest tightness
Radiation	Trapezius ridges	—	—	—	—	Dermatomal pattern	+/- to back	Right scapular tip	—
Associated signs and symptoms	Pericardial rub +/- effusion	—	Acid taste in mouth	—	Cough Fever Dyspnea	Vesicular rash	N/V melena	N/V Anorexia	Sweating Palpitations SOB
Factors that exacerbate	Supine Deep breathing	Swallowing	Eating Supine position	Palpation of affected site	Deep breaths	Palpation of affected area	Meals	Fatty foods	—
Relieving factors	Leaning forward	NTG CCB	Antacids	NSAIDs	Oxygen NSAIDs	Antivirals Steroids	Antacids	NPO	Benzos
Diagnostic studies	ECG 2D-echo ↑ TnI = myo-pericarditis	UGI Esoph. Manometry	EGD pH probe UGI	Clinical diagnosis	CXR Sputum cx Abnormal lung exam	Clinical diagnosis	EGD H. pylori testing	RUQ ultrasound	Diagnosis of exclusion
Therapy	NSAIDs Colchicine Gluco-corticoids	CCB Nitrates	Acid suppression therapy	NSAIDs	Antibiotics Thoracentesis if large effusion	Antivirals Glucocorticoids	PPI; H₂-blocker; +/- H. pylori rx	Surgery	Counseling Anxiolytics

HEART FAILURE (HF)

- **Definition**: HF is a condition during which the heart is unable to deliver sufficient oxygenated blood to meet the metabolic demands of the tissues.
- **Etiologies**: CAD, HTN, valvular cardiomyopathy, myocarditis, infiltrative cardiomyopathy (amyloidosis, hemochromatosis, sarcoidosis), constrictive pericarditis, toxin-induced cardiomyopathy (anthracyclines, alcohol), beriberi, thyrotoxicosis, or peripartum cardiomyopathy
- **Precipitants of acute decompensated heart failure (ADHF)**: MI, cardiac ischemia, ARF, hypertensive crisis, medication or dietary noncompliance, pulmonary disease, anemia, pulmonary embolus, thyroid disease, substance abuse, or arrhythmia

Table 4-8 Staging and Classification of Heart Failure

New York Heart Association (NYHA) classification (current clinical status)		AHA/ACC stages of heart failure (represents **worst** clinical status)	
Class 1	Asymptomatic except with very strenuous activity	Stage A	Risk factors for heart failure present; patient is asymptomatic
Class 2	Symptoms with moderate exertion	Stage B	Asymptomatic; pt has CAD, LVH, valvular heart disease, or LVEF < 0.4
Class 3	Symptoms with activities of daily living	Stage C	Structural heart disease with mild–moderate heart failure
Class 4	Symptoms at rest	Stage D	End-stage heart failure

CAD = coronary artery disease; LVH = left ventricular hypertrophy, LVEF = left ventricular ejection fraction.
Adapted from ACC/AHA Clinical Practice Guidelines on Chronic Heart Failure in *JACC* 2005;46:1116–1143.

- **Clinical presentation**
  - ➤ **Congestion**—left-sided: S_3, pulmonary rales, DOE, orthopnea, and PND; right-sided: JVD, HJR, ascites, and peripheral edema
  - ➤ **Low perfusion/output (forward failure)**—cold extremities, AMS, oliguria, fatigue, pulsus alternans, hypotension, and narrow pulse pressure: (SBP – DBP)/SBP < 25%
- **Initial evaluation**
  - ➤ ECG, chest radiograph, and 2-D echocardiogram
  - ➤ Labs: CBC, CHEM-7, liver and fasting lipid panels, TnI, BNP/NT-proBNP, and oximetry
    - ○ Other causes of ↑ BNP: septic shock, acute PE, ARDS, Cor pulmonale, renal failure (CrCl < 60 mL/min), cirrhosis, thyrotoxicosis, pulmonary hypertension, and subarachnoid hemorrhage
  - ➤ Monitor: strict I's/O's, daily weights, potassium, and BUN/creatinine
- **ADHF therapy**
  - ➤ **Wet/warm** (49%): IV diuretics, oxygen, morphine, and nitrates (SL or cutaneous)
    - ○ Vasodilators if NL/elevated BP and poor response to diuretics and nitrates
    - ○ Consider noninvasive ventilation for moderate–severe HF with respiratory failure

Table 4-9 Clinical Findings in Patients with Suspected Heart Failure

Clinical Finding	Sensitivity	Specificity	Positive LR	Negative LR
Dyspnea on exertion	100%	17%	1.2	0
Paroxysmal nocturnal dyspnea	39%	80%	2	0.8
Prior MI	59%	86%	4.1	0.5
Laterally displaced cardiac apex (PMI)	66%	95%	16	0.4
Dependent edema	20%	86%	1.4	0.9
S_3 gallop	24%	99%	27	0.8
Hepatojugular reflux	33%	94%	6	0.7
Jugular venous distension	17%	98%	9.3	0.8
Pulmonary rales	29%	77%	1.3	0.9
CXR showing cardiomegaly and/or pulmonary edema	71%	92%	8.9	0.3
ECG with anterior Q waves or LBBB	94%	61%	2.4	0.1
BNP > 500 pg/mL	90% PPV for HF			
BNP < 50 pg/mL	98% NPV excluding HF			
BNP < 100 pg/mL	90% NPV excluding HF			
NT-proBNP > 450 pg/mL (<50 yr)	95% PPV for HF			
NT-proBNP > 900 pg/mL (50–75 yr)	95% PPV for HF			
NT-proBNP > 1800 pg/mL (>75 yr)	95% PPV for HF			
NT-proBNP < 300 pg/mL	98% NPV excluding HF			

Adapted from *Am Fam Physician* 2004;70:2145 and *Crit Care Med* 2005;33:2094.

> **Wet/cold** (20%): IV diuretics, oxygen, and vasodilators
>   ○ Consider ICU admission with central hemodynamic monitoring
>   ○ May need inotropic therapy if very low output state
>   ○ Mechanical assist devices for refractory hypotension or low cardiac output: IABP (not if severe AI, sepsis, or recent CVA); LVAD (bridge to transplant)
> **Dry/warm** (27%): decrease chronic diuretic dose or cautious fluid challenge, oxygen, and afterload reduction (ACEI, ARB, or hydralazine plus nitrates)
> **Dry/cold** (4%): cautious fluid challenge, oxygen, and inotropic therapy
>   ○ Consider ICU admission with central hemodynamic monitoring
>   ○ Mechanical assist devices for refractory hypotension or low cardiac output (as above)

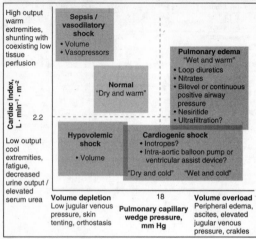

Reprinted with permission from *American Journal of Cardiology*, 2005;96(6A):32G–40G.

Figure 4-3 Classification of Acute Decompensated Heart Failure

- IV loop diuretics: furosemide 20–40 mg, bumetanide 2–4 mg, or torsemide 10–20 mg
  - ➤ Double diuretic dose every 15–20 min until effective diuresis is obtained
- Refractory diuresis
  - ➤ Add thiazide before loop diuretic: chlorothiazide 500 mg IV or metolazone 10 mg PO
  - ➤ Furosemide drip: give bolus dose then start 10–20 mg/hour infusion
  - ➤ Ultrafiltration: use if venous access, SBP > 85 mmHg and no ESRD or shock
- Vasodilators (if BP > 90/60 mmHg)
  - ➤ Nitroglycerin: 5–10 mcg/min to max 200 mcg/min; nitroprusside start 0.3–0.5 mcg/kg/min; nesiritide 2 mcg/kg bolus then 0.01 mcg/kg/min (may ↑ mortality and serum creatinine)
- Inotropes for low-output states (especially if SBP < 85 mmHg or cardiorenal syndrome; watch for ↓↓ BP)
  - ➤ Dobutamine: start at 2.5 mcg/kg/min and titrate to max 20 mcg/kg/min
  - ➤ Milrinone: 50 mcg/kg load over 10 min → 0.2–0.75 mcg/kg/min (causes less tachycardia)
- β-blockers in ADHF
  - ➤ No change to β-blocker dose in wet/warm or dry/warm ADHF
  - ➤ Hold or decrease β-blocker dose 50% in wet/cold or dry/cold ADHF

- Indication for heart transplantation
  - ➤ Refractory CHF, ischemia, or arrhythmias despite optimal medical therapy
  - ➤ Poor candidates: pulmonary hypertension, sepsis, CA, advanced lung disease, cirrhosis, ESRD, substance abuse, age > 60 yr, or noncompliance
- Prognosis in ADHF
  - ➤ CART risk analysis—risk factors (RFs): BUN ≥ 43 mg/dL; crt ≥ 2.75 mg/dL; SBP < 115
    - ○ In-house mortality: 22% if all 3 RFs present; 2% if no RFs present
  - ➤ Pre-discharge BNP: > 700 has 15 × ↑ 6 mo death or readmissions vs < 350 pg/mL
  - ➤ Initial TnI ≥ 1 mcg/L has 8% in-house mortality vs 2.7% if TnI normal

Table 4-10 Stepwise Medication Approach for Chronic HF Therapy

Systolic HF (LVEF ≤ 0.4)	Diastolic HF (LVEF > 0.4)
1. Diuretics for volume control	1. Diuretics for volume control
2. Afterload therapy: ACEI; ARB; or hydralazine plus nitrates	2. BP control: ACEI, ARB, β-blocker, verapamil, or diltiazem
3. β-blocker titrated to HR 55–65	3. Control cardiac ischemia: meds vs revascularization
4. Aldosterone antagonists	
5. Digoxin (<1 ng/mL) for symptom control	4. HR control for Afib/Aflut:
6. Statin may be beneficial	β-blocker, verapamil, or diltiazem

Table 4-11 Nonpharmacological Interventions for HF Management

• 2 g/d sodium restriction	• Weight loss for obese patients
• Maintenance of BP at < 130/80 mmHg	• Fluid restriction: <2 L/day if serum Na < 130 and < 1.5 L/day if serum Na < 125 MEq/L
• Smoking cessation	
• Moderate alcohol consumption	• Education: diet, meds, lifestyle modification

- **Devices to Consider in Chronic HF**
  - ➤ ICD if LVEF ≤0.3 with NYHA ≥class 2 CHF **OR** any history of cardiac arrest, VF, or unstable VT and expected survival more than 1 yr
  - ➤ Biventricular pacemaker if LVEF ≤0.35 and NYHA ≥class 3 CHF on optimal med therapy, QRS duration ≥120 msec, and expected survival more than 1 yr

References: Congestive Heart Failure 2008;14:127; 2008;14:19; J Am Coll Cardiol 2007; 50:2357; Clev Clin J Med 2006;73:557.

ATRIAL FIBRILLATION

Etiologies of Afib (mnemonic is CPR HEARTS)

- **C**—coronary artery disease (CAD) or acute MI
- **P**—pulmonary (COPD/obstructive sleep apnea), pheochromocytoma, and pericarditis
- **R**—rheumatic heart disease (or valvular cardiomyopathy)
- **H**—hypertensive or hypertrophic cardiomyopathy or severe hypoxia
- **E**—embolus (pulmonary)
- **A**—alcohol and amyloidosis
- **R**—ruled out cardiopulmonary disease (if none present, then lone Afib)
- **T**—theophylline toxicity, thyrotoxicosis or trauma (blunt chest)
- **S**—surgery (e.g., post-CABG), sick sinus syndrome, sarcoidosis, or sympathomimetic toxicity

Classification of Afib
- Paroxysmal
- Persistent (converts with electrical/chemical cardioversion)
- Permanent (resistant to electrical/chemical cardioversion)

Workup of Afib
- ECG, chest radiograph, and 2-D echocardiogram
- Labs: CBC, CHEM-7, liver panel, TSH +/− blood alcohol level, and urine drug screen
- Electrophysiologic study (EPS) to determine the etiology of wide-complex tachycardias or for curative atrial or AV nodal ablation in chronic or paroxysmal Afib/Aflut
- Noninvasive testing to rule out cardiac ischemia if clinically indicated

Table 4-12 CHADS$_2$ Score to Determine* the Embolic Risk for Stroke in Nonvalvular Afib

CHADS$_2$ score	Adjusted stroke rate[†]	CHADS$_2$ stroke risk
0	1.9	Low level
1	2.8	Low level
2	4.0	Moderate level
3	5.9	Moderate level
4	8.5	High level
5	12.5	High level
6	18.2	High level

* CHADS$_2$ score = One point each for **C**HF exacerbation in last 100 d, **H**TN, **A**ge > 75 yr, and **D**M; 2 points for history of **S**troke/TIA. Warfarin recommended for CHADS$_2$ ≥ 2; aspirin recommended for CHADS$_2$ 0–1.
† Number of strokes per 100 patient-years from the National Registry of Atrial Fibrillation.
Adapted from *Annals Intern Med* 2003;139:1009–1017.

Antithrombotic Therapy to Minimize Cardioembolic Stroke Risk
- Therapy indicated for persistent, permanent, or recurrent paroxysmal Afib
- Chronic anticoagulation with warfarin titrated to INR 2.5 (range 2–3) indicated for CHADS$_2$ score ≥ 2; valvular Afib; history of prior cardioembolic stroke/TIA; prosthetic heart valve; women ≥ 75 yr; LVEF ≤ 0.35; atrial thrombus; **or** age ≥ 65 yr with DM or CHF
- Aspirin 81–325 mg PO daily if nonvalvular Afib with CHADS$_2$ score ≤1
- In nonvalvular Afib, warfarin reduces stroke risk 64% and aspirin reduces risk 22%
- Warfarin ↑ risk of serious intracranial hemorrhage 0.2%/year versus aspirin
- Warfarin contraindications: fall risk, noncompliance, active drug or alcohol abuse, unstable psychiatric conditions, hemorrhagic diathesis, severe thrombocytopenia, recent neurosurgery, ophthalmologic or trauma surgery, active bleeding, pericarditis, endocarditis, history of intracranial hemorrhage, regional anesthesia, pregnancy, or threatened abortion

AFib Rate Versus Rhythm Control
- Rate control plus antithrombotic therapy is preferred over rhythm control in elderly patients with advanced heart disease.
  ➢ Desired resting rate 60–80 and 90–115 with exercise or during 6-minute walk test
- Consider rhythm control in younger patients with minimal heart disease or for disabling symptoms or poor exercise capacity in those with advanced heart disease.

Table 4-13 Agents for Afib Rate Control

Agent	Acute IV therapy	Chronic oral Rx	Comments
Metoprolol*	5 mg q 5 min × 3	25–100 mg bid	Good for CAD
Esmolol*	500 mcg/kg IVP then 6–200 mcg/kg/min		Caution if ↓ BP, severe bronchospasm, or HF
Diltiazem*	0.25 mg/kg IVP → 5–15 mg/h	120–360 mg daily	Caution if severe HF or hypotension
Verapamil*	2.5–5 mg q 15 min × 2	120–360 mg daily	
Digoxin*	10–15 mcg/kg in divided doses q6h	0.125–0.375 mg daily (if NL renal function)	Use if HF; ↓ dose if CrCl < 50 mL/min
Amiodarone	150 mg over 10 min → 1 mg/min × 6 h → 0.5 mg/min × 18 hr	200–400 mg daily	Good for HF or WPW; Many drug interactions

* Contraindicated if evidence of pre-excitation syndrome or accessory pathway (e.g., WPW); Rx = therapy.
Adapted from *J Am Coll Cardiol* 2006;48:e149–246.

Synchronized Electrical or Chemical Cardioversion
- Timing of electrical or chemical cardioversion
  - ➤ Immediately if hemodynamically unstable (chest pain, CHF, or shock)
  - ➤ If negative transthoracic echocardiogram and Afib duration < 48 hours, *or*
  - ➤ Negative transesophageal echocardiogram and heparin anticoagulation started, *or*
  - ➤ After 3 weeks of adequate warfarin anticoagulation
- Biphasic shock using anterior and posterior placement of pads has the highest rate of successful electrical cardioversion (nearly 100%)
- Medical cardioversion: amiodarone, dofetilide, flecainide, ibutilide, or propafenone
- Avoid cardioversion if Afib > 6 months, left atrium > 5 cm, or endocardial clot present
- Continue warfarin for at least 4 weeks after successful cardioversion
- Continue converting agent × 2 weeks **AND** continue a β-blocker or diltiazem/verapamil after a successful cardioversion to prevent atrial remodeling and to maintain sinus rhythm

Special Circumstances
- Pre-excitation syndrome/accessory pathway
  - ➤ Suggested by ventricular rate > 220, delta waves, or ↑ HR after giving AV nodal blocker
  - ➤ Rate control with amiodarone or ibutilide or DC cardioversion
  - ➤ Eventually, catheter ablation for Afib with an accessory pathway is required
- Acute MI
  - ➤ β-blocker, diltiazem, or verapamil (LVEF > 0.35); amiodarone (LVEF ≤ 0.35)
- Hyperthyroidism
  - ➤ β-blocker and antithyroid medications for rate control
  - ➤ Consider acute anticoagulation depending on comorbid conditions
- Pregnancy
  - ➤ Digoxin, β-blocker, verapamil or diltiazem are safe for rate control
  - ➤ Subcutaneous UFH, LMWH, and aspirin are safe antithrombotic medications
- Tachy-brady syndrome
  - ➤ AV-sequential pacemaker insertion then aggressive AV nodal blocker therapy

- Catheter ablation of atrial focus for refractory symptoms or poor rate control on meds
  - ➤ The Maze procedure is an option during concomitant cardiac surgery

References: J Am Coll Cardiol 2006;48:e149–246; JAMA 2003;290(2):2685–2692; Ann Intern Med 2003;139:1009–1033; NEJM 2001;344:1411–1420; NEJM 2002;347:1825–1840; and Ann Intern Med 2007;146:857–867.

WIDE-COMPLEX TACHYCARDIAS

General Workup
- ECG, echocardiogram, PA/Lat CXR, chemistry panel, and resting oximetry
- Noninvasive stress testing if significant probability of CAD or for any exercise-induced VT
- Continuous cardiac monitoring

Table 4-14 Ventricular Tachycardia Versus SVT with Aberrancy

Factors Favoring Ventricular Tachycardia	Factors Favoring SVT with Aberrancy
• AV dissociation	• Preexisting bundle branch block (BBB)
• Fusion beats	• Known pre-excitation syndrome
• Capture beats	• Preceding atrial activity
• Concordance of precordial QRS complexes	• Initial beat PAC with narrow QRS complex
• Structurally abnormal heart*	• Structurally normal heart
• Essentially regular rhythm	• BBB alternating with normal beats
• QRS duration > 0.14 msec	• Initial deflection in same direction as QRS complexes
• Marked RUQ axis deviation	
• QRS morphology: monophasic R wave, qR, or Rsr, in V_1 or MCL	• QRS morphology: rSR, or RSR, in V_1 or MCL

* History of MI, CHF, hypertensive or hypertrophic cardiomyopathy, or LVEF < 0.4.

Management of VT
- Correct any abnormal electrolytes and discontinue all offending drugs
- Treat all wide-complex tachycardias (WCTs) initially as VT until etiology firmly established
- Structurally abnormal heart
  - ➤ LVEF ≤ 0.35 and NYHA ≥ 2 HF on meds or history of sustained VT/VF → ICD placement
  - ➤ Known CAD or significant cardiac ischemia by noninvasive testing → revascularization
  - ➤ LVEF > 0.35 and nonischemic cardiomyopathy → β-blocker therapy
- Normal heart
  - ➤ Sustained VT → cardiac catheterization +/− electrophysiological study (EPS)
  - ➤ NSVT and significant ischemia by noninvasive testing → cardiac catheterization +/− EPS
  - ➤ NSVT and no cardiac ischemia by noninvasive testing → β-blocker therapy
  - ➤ Right ventricular outflow tract VT suggested by normal resting ECG and LBBB-type VT with inferior QRS axis → ICD for history of sustained VT/VF
- Antiarrhythmic therapy indicated for recurrent VT: use β-blockers, amiodarone, or sotalol (if normal left ventricular systolic function)

Management of Polymorphic VT
- Torsades de pointes if prolonged QTc: discontinue all offending meds and treat with magnesium sulfate 4 g IV
  ➤ Pacemaker indicated for torsades de pointes 2° to heart block or symptomatic bradycardia
- Brugada syndrome: atypical RBBB; ST elevation in V_1; absence of deep S in I, aVL, or V_6
  ➤ ICD for previous cardiac arrest on optimal meds and select pts who have had syncope

Indication for Electrophysiological Testing
- In patients with CAD to determine etiology of WCT or to assess efficacy of VT ablation
- Diagnosis of bundle branch reentrant tachycardia and to guide ablation
- Evaluation of WCT if nonischemic cardiomyopathy and palpitations, presyncope, or syncope

Indications for Radiofrequency Ablation
- Patients with an ICD in place who have drug-resistant VT or are intolerant of medications
- Bundle branch reentrant VT or right ventricular outflow tract reentrant VT
- Afib with Wolff-Parkinson-White (WPW) or a history of sudden cardiac arrest
Reference: J Am Coll Cardiol 2006;48:1064.

INDICATIONS FOR PACEMAKERS AND DEFIBRILLATORS

ACC/AHA Indications for Pacemaker Insertion
- **Symptomatic bradycardia:** any documented bradyarrhythmia that is directly responsible for the development of syncope, near syncope, lightheadedness, or transient confusional states from cerebral hypoperfusion
- **Pacing for acquired atrioventricular (AV) block**
  ➤ **Reversible causes of AV block have been ruled out** (e.g., MI or abnormal electrolytes)
  ➤ Type II second-degree AV block (especially if a wide QRS or symptoms are present)
  ➤ Third-degree AV block (complete heart block [CHB]), excluding congenital CHB
  ➤ Can consider for first-degree AV block (PR > 0.30 sec) or type I second-degree AV block with symptomatic bradycardia
- **Pacing for chronic bifascicular or trifascicular block**
  ➤ If ambulatory ECG monitoring reveals intermittent type II second-degree AV block or third-degree AV block
- **Pacing in sinus node dysfunction**
  ➤ Symptomatic sinus pauses (≥3 sec)
  ➤ Symptomatic chronotropic incompetence
- **Pacing in carotid sinus syndrome and neurocardiogenic syncope**
  ➤ Documented asystole > 3 sec with minimal carotid sinus pressure
  ➤ Recurrent neurocardiogenic syncope associated with bradycardia
- **Pacing in tachy-brady syndrome**
  ➤ Pacemaker inserted to prevent symptomatic bradycardia when AV nodal blocking agents used to rate control rapid Afib/Aflut
- **Indications for atrial overdrive pacing to terminate tachyarrhythmias**

> If unresponsive to antiarrhythmic therapy; and atrial overdrive pacing useful for symptomatic, recurrent supraventricular tachycardia that is terminated by pacing

Pacemaker Tips
- Chronic ventricular pacing can lead to ventricular dyssynchrony and increase the risk of CHF. Attempt to adjust pacemaker to maximize atrial pacing and minimize ventricular pacing (i.e., set a slow backup ventricular rate and a long PR interval).

Indications for Implantable Cardioverter-Defibrillator (ICD) Insertion
- Symptomatic sustained VT or VF
- Nonsustained VT with CAD and left ventricular systolic dysfunction (LVEF < 0.4)
- Ischemic/nonischemic cardiomyopathy (LVEF ≤ 0.3) and refractory NYHA 2–3 CHF
- Life expectancy is at least 1 yr

Indications for Biventricular (BiV) Pacing/Cardiac Resynchronization Therapy
- Medically refractory NYHA class 3–4 CHF with LVEF ≤ 35%, sinus rhythm, QRS ≥ 120 msec, and a life expectancy of at least 1 yr

Pacemaker Follow-Up via Transtelephonic or Office Monitoring
- Check pacemaker at 6 weeks after implantation, then every 6 months until battery power starts to fall, then every 3 months until battery power is at the elective replacement level.
- Check the function of an ICD or biventricular pacer every 3 months.

References: J Am Coll Cardiol 2002;40(9):1703–1719; 2004;43(2):1145–1148.

ACUTE PERICARDITIS

Etiologies
- Excluding patients with known CA, ESRD, trauma, and postradiation, 90% of cases are idiopathic or of viral etiology
- Other causes: neoplastic, infectious (tuberculous, bacterial, fungal, rickettsial, or fungal), Dressler's syndrome (post-MI), postradiation, chest trauma, uremia, postpericardiotomy, hypothyroidism, connective tissue diseases (systemic lupus erythematosus, scleroderma, and rheumatoid arthritis), and meds (hydralazine, isoniazid, methyldopa, phenytoin, and procainamide)

Clinical Presentation
- Sudden onset of constant, sharp, or stabbing, retrosternal chest pain
- Exacerbating factors: deep inspiration, lying down, and possibly with swallowing
- Alleviating factors: improved with leaning forward
- Radiation pattern: neck, arms, shoulders, trapezius muscle ridges, or epigastrium
- Classically, there is no improvement with nitroglycerin
- Associated symptoms: malaise, myalgias, dry cough, and dyspnea are common

Physical Exam
- Pericardial rub in 85% of patients: harsh, high-pitched, scratchy sound best heard at end expiration with the patient leaning forward using the stethoscope's diaphragm
  > Classic rub with 3 components best heard at the apex: ventricular systole, early diastole, and atrial systole. 50% of rubs triphasic, 33% biphasic, and the rest monophasic
- Signs of cardiac tamponade: muffled heart sounds, hypotension, tachycardia, jugular venous distension, and pulsus paradoxus (fall in systolic blood pressure >10 mmHg with inspiration)
- Temperature > 38°C uncommon except in purulent pericarditis

Electrocardiographic Changes (seen in 90% of patients)
- **Stage 1**: Diffuse, **upward concave** ST-segment elevations and PR-segment depressions in all leads (especially leads I, II, aVL, aVF, and V_3–V_6), except lead aVR where ST-segment depression and PR-segment elevation occurs. No T-wave inversions.
- **Stage 2**: ST and PR segments normalize and T waves progressively flatten
- **Stage 3**: Diffuse T-wave inversions
- **Stage 4**: Normalization of the T waves
- Electrical alternans may be seen if a large pericardial effusion exists
- A ratio of ST-segment elevation (in mm) to T-wave amplitude (in mm) greater than 0.24 in lead V_6 is highly specific for acute pericarditis
- Diffuse T-wave inversions **AND** concave ST ↑ and PR ↓ suggests myopericarditis

Prognostic Factors Warranting Admission to Hospital
- Fever > 38°C, subacute onset over weeks, immunocompromised, history of trauma, anticoagulant therapy, myocarditis, elevated troponin I, evidence of cardiac tamponade, or a large pericardial effusion (echo-free space > 2 cm)

Workup of Acute Pericarditis
- Labs: complete blood count, renal panel, troponin I +/− ANA (antinuclear antibody) +/− RF (rheumatoid factor) +/− PPD (positive purified derivative test)
- If tuberculous or malignant effusion suspected, pericardial fluid should be sent for cytology, CEA (level ≥ 5 ng/mL is 75% sensitive and 100% specific for malignancy) and *Mycobacterium tuberculosis* RNA by polymerase chain reaction assay and adenosine deaminase activity (>30 units/L suggests tuberculous pericarditis)
- Chest radiograph
- Echocardiogram is indicated in all patients with suspected pericarditis

Treatment of Acute Pericarditis
- Oral indomethacin 75–225 mg/day or ibuprofen 1600–3200 mg/day
  ➤ Colchicine 0.6 mg PO bid can be added if symptoms persist >2 weeks or for recurrent pericarditis and continue 0.6 mg PO daily–bid for up to 6 months
- Prednisone 1–1.5 mg/kg/day orally × 1 month then taper over several months only for severe, recurrent pericarditis or if due to a connective tissue disease or for tuberculous pericarditis
- Avoid all anticoagulants if possible as they increase the risk of a hemopericardium
- Pericardiocentesis: therapeutic for clinical evidence of tamponade or diagnostic for possible tuberculous, bacterial, or neoplastic pericarditis
  ➤ Fluid for cell count, culture, Gram stain, protein, LDH, glucose +/− cytology
- Pericardial window or pericardiectomy for recurrent large effusions

Reference: NEJM 2004;351;21:2195; Lancet 2004;351:2195; and Circulation 2003;108:1146–1162.

VALVULAR HEART DISEASE: AORTIC STENOSIS

Clinical Presentation
- Chest pain (angina), dyspnea (heart failure), or exertional syncope

Exam
- Harsh, crescendo–decrescendo systolic murmur at right 2nd intercostal space → carotids
- Soft aortic component of S_2 (A_2)
- Gallavardin sign
- Markers of severe AS: late-peaking, long murmur, S_4 gallop, sustained PMI, weak and delayed carotid pulse (pulsus parvus et tardus)

Table 4-15 Echocardiographic Features of Aortic Stenosis

Characteristic	Mild AS	Moderate AS	Severe AS
Mean gradient (mmHg)	<25	25–40	>40*
Valve area (cm²)	>1.5	1–1.5	<1†
Jet velocity (m/sec)	<3	3–4	>4

* If left ventricular ejection fraction <0.4, may have severe AS with only a moderate gradient of 25–40 mmHg.
† Valve area index (cm² per m²) < 0.6 also indicates severe AS.
Adapted from J Am Coll Cardiol 2008;52 e1–e142.

Indications for Cardiac Catheterization
- Prior to an AVR, to assess for CAD in patients at risk or if considering a pulmonary allograft
- To assess severity of AS when noninvasive studies are inconclusive or not consistent with clinical findings

Medical Therapy
- Indicated primarily to bridge patients until they have an AVR
- Heart failure
  > Mild–moderate: judicious diuretics; control BP with ACEI; and digoxin for LVEF < 0.4
  > Severe HF with a normal BP and LVEF ≤ 0.35: nitroprusside with central hemodynamic monitoring titrated to MAP 60–70 mmHg
- Afib: digoxin for ventricular rate control
- Angina: cautious use of β-blockers and nitrates

Indications for Surgical Treatment
- AVR for severe aortic stenosis and any of the following:
  > Undergoing CABG or other heart surgery (may also consider AVR for moderate AS)
  > Presence of CHF, angina, or syncope
  > LVEF < 0.5
  > Consider for hypotension during a supervised exercise test
- Aortic balloon valvotomy reasonable option for:
  > Hemodynamically unstable or pregnant patients with severe AS at high risk for an AVR
  > Palliation for severe AS in patients who are not candidates for an AVR

References: J Am Coll Cardiol 2008;52:e1 and NEJM 2003;348:1756.

VALVULAR HEART DISEASE: AORTIC INSUFFICIENCY

Clinical Presentation
- Acute AI presents with heart failure +/− hypotension or cardiogenic shock
- Chronic AI presents with heart failure

Exam
- Blowing, decrescendo diastolic murmur at LSB (valve disorder) or RSB (aortic root disorder); increased during expiration and with a strong handgrip
- Additional signs: low diastolic blood pressure, bisferiens pulse (double pulse) of carotids; water hammer carotid pulse (Corrigan); femoral bruits (Duroziez); head bob (de Musset); pulsation of the uvula (Müller); and subungual pulsations (Quincke)
- Indicators of severity in chronic AI: wide pulse pressure with a low diastolic blood pressure, Austin Flint murmur (diastolic rumble at apex), long duration of murmur, S_3 gallop, a laterally displaced and wide PMI, and a soft S_1

Workup
- Echocardiogram: severe AI with Doppler jet width > 65% left ventricular outflow tract and vena contracta width > 0.6, LV systolic diameter > 55 mm, or LV diastolic diameter > 75 mm
- Radionuclide ventriculography or cardiac MRI if LV function equivocal by echocardiogram
- Cardiac catheterization indicated if noninvasive tests are equivocal or discordant with clinical symptoms, or to evaluate for CAD in patients at risk
  - ➤ Severe AI if regurgitant volume ≥ 60 mL/beat, regurgitant fraction ≥ 50%, regurgitant orifice area ≥ 0.3 cm^2, and/or dilated left ventricle

Medical Treatment
- Vasodilators (ACEI, nifedipine ER, amlodipine, felodipine, or hydralazine) for severe chronic AI or LVEF < 0.4
- Loop diuretics indicated for volume control in CHF
- Acute severe AI: nitroprusside +/– dobutamine or dopamine as bridge to urgent AVR
  - ➤ Intra-aortic balloon pump and vasoconstrictors are contraindicated.

Indications for AVR
- Symptomatic severe AI
- LVEF ≤ 0.5
- Left ventricular end-systolic dimension > 55 mm or end-diastolic dimension > 75 mm
- Severe AI in patients undergoing a CABG or other surgery on the heart or aorta
References: J Am Coll Cardiol 2008;52:e1; NEJM 2004;351:1539; and NEJM 2005;353:1342.

VALVULAR HEART DISEASE: MITRAL STENOSIS (MS)

Clinical Presentation
- Heart failure, palpitations (Afib), stroke, or pulmonary hypertension

Exam
- Diastolic rumble at apex with presystolic accentuation (if sinus rhythm); opening snap; ↑ S_1
- Indicators of severity: long duration of murmur and shorter S_2 → opening snap interval

Table 4-16 Echocardiographic Features of Mitral Stenosis

Characteristic	Mild MS	Moderate MS	Severe MS
Mean gradient (mmHg)	<5	5–10	>10
Pulmonary artery systolic pressure (mmHg)	<30	30–50	>50
Valve area (cm^2)	>1.5	1–1.5	<1

Adapted from *JACC* 2008;52:e1.

Indications for Cardiac Catheterization
- Noninvasive testing is equivocal or discordant with clinical symptoms
- Hemodynamic evaluation when echo reveals discrepancy between MV gradient and MV area
- To assess cause of pulmonary hypertension when noninvasive testing is inconclusive

Medical Therapy
- Afib: anticoagulation with heparin/warfarin; rate control with digoxin, β-blocker, verapamil or diltiazem; DC cardioversion for severe hemodynamic instability

- Heart failure: sodium restriction, judicious diuresis, Afib rate control, and avoid tachycardia
- Chronic anticoagulation if: chronic or paroxysmal Afib/Aflut, prior embolization, severe MS with a left atrium (LA) > 5.5 cm or presence of an LA clot

Surgical Therapy
- Indications for percutaneous mitral balloon valvulotomy (PMBV)
  - ➤ Moderate–severe MS with NYHA class II–IV CHF
  - ➤ Moderate–severe MS and pulmonary artery systolic pressure >50 mmHg (rest) or > 60 (exercise)
- Contraindications for PMBV: LA clot, moderate–severe MR, or MV morphology not suitable
- Indications for MV replacement or repair
  - ➤ Moderate–severe MS with NYHA class III–IV CHF and PMBV unavailable or contraindicated
  - ➤ Moderate–severe MS with NYHA class I–II CHF and pulmonary artery systolic pressure >60 mmHg in noncandidates for PMBV

References: J Am Coll Cardiol 2008;52:e1 and Circulation 2005;112:432.

VALVULAR HEART DISEASE: MITRAL REGURGITATION (MR)

Clinical Presentation
- Heart failure, palpitations (Afib), stroke, or pulmonary hypertension
- Acute MR can present with CHF and hypotension or cardiogenic shock

Exam
- Blowing, systolic murmur at apex → left axilla; ↑ with strong handgrip; ↓ with valsalva
- Soft S_1 and may have an S_3 gallop or laterally displaced and enlarged PMI

Table 4-17 Echocardiographic Features of Mitral Regurgitation (MR)

Characteristics	Mild MR	Moderate MR	Severe MR
Doppler jet area	<20% LA area	20–40% LA area	>40% LA area*
Doppler vena contracta width	<0.3 cm	0.3–0.69 cm	>0.7 cm

* Severe MR also if any LA swirling or if jet impinges on LA wall.
Adapted from *JACC* 2008;52:e1.

Indications for Cardiac Catheterization
- LV hemodynamic evaluation when echocardiogram is equivocal or discordant with clinical findings or displays a discrepancy between MR severity and ↑ pulmonary artery pressures
- Evaluate for CAD in patients at risk

Medical Therapy
- Heart failure: sodium restriction, diuretics, nitrates, and afterload reduction (ACEI, ARB, or hydralazine/nitrates); add β-blocker if LVEF < 0.4
- Afib: anticoagulation with heparin/warfarin; rate control with digoxin, β-blocker, verapamil, or diltiazem; DC cardioversion for severe hemodynamic instability
- Acute MR with normal BP: nitroprusside with central hemodynamic monitoring
- Acute MR with hypotension: nitroprusside and dobutamine +/– IABP → urgent MVR

Indications for Mitral Valve Repair or Replacement
- Acute symptomatic severe MR
- Chronic severe MR with NYHA class II–IV CHF and:

> LVEF 0.3–0.6 and/or LV end-systolic dimension (LVESD) ≥ 40 mm
> Consider if LVEF > 0.6, LVESD < 40 mm, and new-onset Afib or pulmonary HTN

References: J Am Coll Cardiol 2008;52:e1; NEJM 2004;351:1627; and Circulation 2003; 108:2432.

HYPERTENSION

Table 4-18 Risk Stratification for Hypertensive Patients

Risk factors	End-organ damage
Cigarette smoking	Heart disease
Obesity (body mass index ≥ 30 kg/m²)	• Left ventricular hypertrophy
Family history of cardiovascular disease: women < 65 yr or men < 55 yr	• Coronary artery disease • Congestive heart failure
Dyslipidemia	Stroke or transient ischemic attack
Diabetes mellitus	Nephropathy (microalbuminuria or
Very sedentary lifestyle	creatinine clearance < 60 mL/min)
Age > 55 yr (men) or > 65 yrs (women)	Peripheral vascular disease
Men or postmenopausal women	Retinopathy

Therapeutic Lifestyle Changes (TLC)
• Weight reduction (aiming for BMI < 25 kg/m²): decreases SBP 5–20 mmHg
• <2 drinks of alcohol/d (men) and ≤1 drink/d (women): decreases SBP 2–4 mmHg
• Aerobic exercise (≥30 min/d ≥ 4 d/wk): decreases SBP 4–9 mmHg
• <2.3 g sodium/d: decreases SBP 2–8 mmHg
• Diet: Dietary Approaches to Stop Hypertension (DASH) diet (↓ SBP 8–14 mmHg); adequate potassium, magnesium, calcium; low saturated fat, high fiber, and low cholesterol
• Smoking cessation

Medications/Herbs That Cause Elevated Blood Pressure (discontinue if possible)
• Anabolic steroids and corticosteroids, bevacizumab, bromocriptine, bupropion, buspirone, clozapine, cyclosporine, darbepoetin, ephedra, epoetin-alpha, estrogens, fludrocortisone, MAOIs, metoclopramide, nicotine, NSAIDs, phentermine, pseudoephedrine, sibutramine, sorafenib, sunitinib, sympathomimetics, tacrolimus, and venlafaxine; herbs: aniseed, bayberry, blue cohosh, capsaicin, ephedra, gentian, ginger, ginseng, guarana, licorice, ma huang, Pau d'Arco, parsley, and St. John's wort

Clinical Conditions That Can Cause Elevated Blood Pressure in Hospitalized Patients
• Important to exclude and address these causes of blood pressure elevation: pain, anxiety, alcohol/drug withdrawal, elevated intracranial pressure, renal failure, excess sodium administration (watch IV fluids), or excessive bladder or bowel distension

Initial Drug Therapy for Uncomplicated Hypertension
• BP goals: BP ≤ 130/80 for DM, CAD, or CKD; BP ≤ 125/75 for proteinuria > 1 g/d
• Initial therapy in patients with no compelling indications for specific drug classes
> Thiazides (drug of choice for most patients if creatinine < 2 mg/dL or CrCl > 35 mL/min/1.73 m²), despite the small increased risk in new-onset diabetes
> Alternative options are: ACEI, CCBs, and ARBs (if ACEI-intolerant)
> β-blockers not the best monotherapy for HTN if no compelling indications
> Stage 2 hypertension usually requires at least 2 drugs

Table 4-19 Compelling Indications for Specific Antihypertensive Drug Therapy

Indication	Drug class
Diabetes with proteinuria	ACEI*, ARB*, verapamil, or diltiazem
Congestive heart failure	ACEI*, ARB*, ß-blockers, diuretics, or AA
Diastolic dysfunction	ß-blocker, verapamil, diltiazem, thiazides, or ACEI*
Isolated systolic hypertension	Thiazides, dihydropyridine CCB, ß-blocker, ACEI*, or nitrates
Post-myocardial infarction	ß-blocker, ACEI*, or AA
Angina	ß-blocker or calcium channel blocker
Atrial fibrillation	ß-blocker, verapamil, or diltiazem
Dyslipidemia	ACEI, ß-blocker, or thiazides
Essential tremor	ß-blocker
Hyperthyroidism	ß-blocker
Migraine	ß-blocker, verapamil, or diltiazem
Osteoporosis	Thiazides
Pregnancy	Methyldopa, hydralazine or labetalol
Benign prostatic hyperplasia	α_1-blockers† in combination with other agents
Erectile dysfunction	ACEI, ARB, or CCB
Renal insufficiency	ACEI* or ARB*
Cerebrovascular disease	Thiazides, ACEI, ARB, or amlodipine
Obstructive sleep apnea	CPAP therapy; AA, thiazides, or CCB at bedtime
African American race	Thiazides (1st line), CCB, or ACEI*
Aortic dissection	Labetalol, ß-blocker, or diltiazem
Refractory hypertension	Minoxidil and loop diuretic and ß-blocker or CCB

AA = aldosterone antagonist; ACEI = angiotensin converting enzyme inhibitor; CCB = calcium channel blocker; ARB = angiotensin receptor blocker; CPAP = continuous positive airway pressure.
* Caution with ACEI or ARB use if creatinine > 3 mg/dL.
† Never use as monotherapy for HTN.

Treatment of Hypertensive Urgency (BP > 180/110 mmHg without end-organ damage)

- Need to exclude chronic, poorly controlled hypertension (outpatient management)
- Oral agents titrated to effect: clonidine 0.2 mg × 1 then 0.1 mg q1h × 6; captopril 25 mg q1h × 4; labetalol 200–400 mg q2–3h; or nifedipine XL 30 mg × 1
- IV agents if pt NPO: metoprolol 5 mg q 15 min × 3; labetalol 20–40 mg q 10–15 min (max 300 mg/d); hydralazine 5–10 mg q 30 min; enalaprilat 1.25 mg q6h; diltiazem 20 mg → 5–15 mg/hr

Initial Workup for Hypertension

- Blood work: Complete blood count, electrolytes, calcium, fasting lipid, and renal panels
- Other studies: urinalysis, ECG, eye exam, and a CXR if signs of CHF
- Eval for secondary HTN if: onset < 30 yr or > 60 yr; accelerated, resistant, or paroxysmal HTN; abnormal UA or ↑ creatinine; unprovoked ↓ K or ↑ Ca; Cushing syndrome; abdominal mass/bruit

Table 4-20 Causes of Secondary Hypertension

Features of secondary hypertension	Possible etiologies
Sudden onset of severe hypertension or newly diagnosed in those <30 yr or >60 yr	Renal vascular disease or renal parenchymal disease
Abnormal urinalysis	Renal parenchymal/glomerular disease
Hypokalemia and ARR >66.9 ng/dL*	Primary hyperaldosteronism
Hypercalcemia	Hyperparathyroidism
Fine tremor, heat intolerance, ↓ TSH, ↑ fT₄	Hyperthyroidism
Paroxysmal severe HTN, palpitations, HA	Pheochromocytoma
Abdominal mass	Polycystic kidney disease
Flank bruit	Renal artery stenosis
↑ glucose, striae, truncal obesity, etc.	Cushing syndrome
Resistant hypertension on three meds	Renal vascular/parenchymal disease
Markedly decreased femoral pulses	Coarctation of aorta
Central obesity, loud snoring, daytime hypersomnolence, nonrestorative sleep	Obstructive sleep apnea

* ARR = aldosterone/renin ratio after 30 minutes sitting > 66.9 ng/dL confirms with 100% specificity, and ARR < 23.6 ng/dL excludes 97% of cases of primary aldosteronism.

Table 4-21 Mechanism of Action of Various Antihypertensive Medications

Diuretics	Negative inotropic	Sympatho-lytics	Renin-angiotensin-aldosterone blockers	Vasodilators
• Furosemide (preferred over thiazides if serum creatinine ≥ 2.5 mg/dL)	• β-blockers • Verapamil • Diltiazem	• β-blockers • Clonidine • Methyl-dopa • Guanethi-dine	• β-blockers • ARBs • ACEIs • Direct renin inhibitors • AAs	• Hydralazine • α₁-blockers • Minoxidil • Dihydropyridine CCBs • Thiazides (creatinine < 2.5 mg/dL)

References: JAMA 2003;289:2560; NEJM 2003;348:610; JAMA 2002;288:2981; J Clin Hypertension 2007;9:10; Circulation 2007;115:2761.

AORTIC DISSECTION

Clinical Presentation
- Acute onset of sharp or tearing anterior chest pain radiating to interscapular area
- Clinicians suspect aortic dissection when present only 15–43% of the time
- Associated signs: diastolic murmur (AI, 31.6%); pulse deficit (15.1–38%); focal neurologic deficits (stroke, 4.7–17%); paraplegia (3–5%); acute limb ischemia (6–28%); acute MI (3.2%); and cardiac tamponade (4–25%)
- Associated symptoms: syncope (8–13%); dyspnea (HF from acute AI, 3–9%); and abdominal pain (mesenteric ischemia, 3.7%)

Risk Factors
- Age > 50 yr, HTN, bicuspid aortic valve, Marfan syndrome, Ehlers-Danlos syndrome, Turner syndrome, giant cell arteritis, syphilitic aortitis, pregnancy, coarctation of aorta, adult polycystic kidney disease, Behçet disease, Takayasu arteritis, blunt chest trauma, cardiac or aortic surgery, or cardiac catheterization

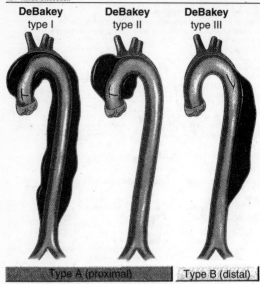

DeBakey type I   **DeBakey type II**   **DeBakey type III**

Type A (proximal)   Type B (distal)

Stanford Classification System

Adapted from Braunwald E. *Heart Disease: A Textbook of Cardiovascular Medicine.* 7th ed. Philadelphia: Elsevier; 2005:1416.

Figure 4-4 Classification System for Aortic Dissection

Workup
- Chest x-ray: widened mediastinum in 44–80% and abnormal aortic contour (56–84%)
- CT scan of aorta with IV contrast (95% sensitivity, 90% specificity)
- MRI with contrast (98% sensitivity, 98% specificity)
- Catheter aortogram (90% sensitivity, 95% specificity)
- Transesophageal echocardiogram (98% sensitivity, 91% specificity)
- Labs: chemistry panel, CBC, PT, PTT, TnI, and ECG

Treatment of Acute Aortic Dissection
- Labetalol or esmolol drip titrated to keep SBP ≤ 110 mmHg and HR < 60 bpm
- Nitroprusside drip can be added for blood pressure control if necessary
- Surgical repair or endovascular treatment indicated for all Stanford type A AD patients
- Endovascular and med treatment preferred for appropriate Stanford type B AD patients

References: JAMA 2000;283:897; Arch Intern Med 2006;166:1350; Circulation 2008;118:S167; Eur J Vasc Endovasc Surg 2006;31:115; and Emerg Clin N Amer 2005;23:1159.

PERIPHERAL ARTERIAL DISEASE (PAD)

Acute Arterial Insufficiency
- Most common cause is a cardioembolic event
- Ischemic complication rate ↑↑ if time from symptom onset to embolectomy is > 6 hr:
  - ➢ 10% if interval < 6 hr; 20% if interval 8 hr; and 33% if interval 24 hr
- Clinical features of arterial insufficiency (6 P's)
  - ➢ Pain, pallor, pulseless, paresthesias, paralysis, and poikilothermia (cold)
  - ➢ Sudden onset of symptoms favors an embolic event
- Treatment
  - ➢ Therapeutic IV heparin then catheter-directed thrombolysis or embolectomy

Chronic Arterial Insufficiency
- Clinical features of PAD
  - ➢ Intermittent claudication described as cramping discomfort, pain, or fatigue of muscles with ambulation (graded by distance walked) and relieved by rest
  - ➢ Aortoiliac disease: thigh/buttock claudication +/− impotence (Leriche syndrome)
  - ➢ Femoropopliteal disease: thigh and calf claudication
  - ➢ Tibial or peroneal artery disease: foot claudication
  - ➢ Signs: dystrophic nails, bruits, absent/weak peripheral pulses, loss of hair on and cold distal extremity, shiny skin, dependent rubor, decreased capillary refill
- Risk Factors: tobacco smoking, positive family history, hyperlipidemia, diabetes, hypertension, hyperhomocysteinemia, and age ≥ 50 yr
- PAD pts: 60–80% have significant CAD and 25% have significant carotid artery stenosis
- PAD pts: 5-year combined event rate of MI, stroke, or vascular death is 35–50%.

Evaluation of PAD

Table 4-22 Ankle-Brachial Index (ABI) to Assess for Lower Extremity PAD

ABI	Interpretation
≥1.3	Noncompressible vessel
0.91–1.29	Normal
0.61–0.9	Mild PAD
0.41–0.6	Moderate PAD
≤0.4	Severe PAD

- Conditions with falsely elevated ABI (usually ABI > 1.3): DM, very elderly, and CKD
  - ➢ Toe-brachial index < 0.7 suggests significant PAD in these patients
- Duplex ultrasound of arterial system and segmental limb pressures: good noninvasive studies to estimate degree of lower extremity arterial obstruction

- Catheter angiogram, CT angiogram, or MR angiogram with 3-D reconstruction all perform well to assess for aortic and/or lower/upper extremity arterial stenoses
- Complete blood count, fasting lipid profile, basic metabolic panel, and ECG
- Consider renal artery imaging to rule out RAS if resistant HTN or renal bruit present

Medical Treatment of PAD

- Lifestyle modification: smoking cessation and graded aerobic exercise program 30 min, 3×/wk
- Lipid control with a statin: LDL < 100 mg/dL (possibly < 70 mg/dL in very high-risk patient*); triglycerides < 150 mg/dL; and HDL > 40 mg/dL
- Tight diabetic (glycohemoglobin < 7%) and blood pressure control (BP < 130/80)
- Aspirin 75–325 mg PO daily (alternative is clopidogrel 75 mg PO daily)
- Cilostazol 100 mg PO bid can improve claudication symptoms and exercise capacity, and is superior to pentoxifylline (avoid if symptoms or history of CHF)
- Pentoxifylline 400 mg PO tid (alternative to cilostazol) modestly ↑ exercise capacity
- β-blockers and ACEI protect against cardiovascular events in these patients
- No benefit of warfarin to ↓ reocclusion rates of arterial grafts or to ↓ claudication

Surgical Treatment or Percutaneous Interventional Therapies for PAD

- Arterial bypass or endovascular revascularization of LE PAD indicated for disabling claudication, rest pain, gangrene, Leriche syndrome, or nonhealing, ischemic ulcers
  ➤ Angioplasty: ↑ success in proximal, large arteries with localized stenosis < 10 cm
  ➤ Surgery preferred if multiple, diffuse stenoses; complete occlusion of artery; bilateral iliac or femoral arteries or aortoiliac disease; or aneurysm surgery also needed
    ○ Grafts – 5-year patency: aortobifem (90%); fem-pop (80%); infrapopliteal (60%)
- Indications for angioplasty subclavian/brachiocephalic arteries: UE claudication; subclavian steal; subclavian stenosis > 50% AND ipsilateral dialysis shunt; before CABG with LIMA to LAD

*Known CAD or CAD risk equivalent and additional risk factors.

References: Circulation 2006;113:e463; JAMA 2006; 295: 547; J Am Coll Cardiol; 2007;50:473; Circulation 2007;116:2203.

SYNCOPE

Table 4-23 Causes of Syncope

Neurally mediated	Orthostatic hypotension	Cardiac arrhythmias	Structural cardiopulmonary	Cerebro-vascular
• Vasovagal • Carotid sinus syndrome • Situational*	• Drug-induced • Autonomic failure[†] • Hypovolemia	• Sick sinus syndrome • AV block • SVT, VT/VF • Pacemaker malfunction	• Acute MI • Aortic stenosis • Pulmonary embolus • Obstructive cardiomyopathy	• Subclavian steal syndrome • Vertebrobasilar TIA • Basilar migraine
66%	10%	11%	5%	1%
Unexplained syncope = 2% and nonsyncopal causes[‡] = 5%				

* Cough, micturition, defecation, swallowing, or postprandial precipitants.
† Shy-Drager syndrome or secondary to amyloidosis, diabetes, Parkinson disease, alcoholism.
‡ Hypoglycemia, hyperventilation, seizures, cataplexy, drop attacks, or psychogenic "pseudo-syncope."
SVT = supraventricular tachycardia; VT = ventricular tachycardia; VF = ventricular fibrillation.
Adapted from Eur Heart J 2006;27:78–82.

History and Exam

- Neurally mediated (can be diagnosed with tilt-table testing in equivocal cases)
  - ➤ Supporting features: absence of cardiac disease; or a long history of recurrent syncope
  - ➤ Precipitating event: fear, pain, unpleasant sight, sound or smell, venipuncture, prolonged standing, or crowded and hot environment
  - ➤ Prodromal symptoms: feeling hot, nausea, lightheadedness, diaphoresis, and visual changes
- Carotid sinus hypersensitivity with head rotation or pressure on lateral neck
  - ➤ Carotid massage (positive with ↓ SBP ≥ 50 mmHg or asystole ≥ 3 sec)
- Orthostatic hypotension
  - ➤ Check for orthostasis (↓ ≥ 20 mmHg SBP, ↑ HR 10–20 from supine to standing)
  - ➤ Autonomic nervous system failure: amyloidosis, diabetes, alcoholism, Parkinson disease, or Shy-Drager syndrome
  - ➤ Syncope occurring within 2 min of standing is suggestive of orthostasis
- Cardiac syncope
  - ➤ Has structural heart disease (CAD, valvular/HTN/hypertrophic cardiomyopathy)
  - ➤ Exertion-related, occurring at rest or in supine location, family history of sudden death or associated with chest discomfort, palpitations, or dyspnea
- Subclavian steal syndrome
  - ➤ Occurs with arm activity; difference > 10 mmHg in systolic BP between arms
- Situational syncope: cough, micturition, or defecation-induced syncope
- Neuropsychiatric: seizures, vertebrobasilar insufficiency, or a conversion disorder
  - ➤ Seizures often have postictal period for > 2 min, tongue biting, tonic-clonic activity, and incontinence

Diagnostic Evaluation

- Hospitalize if: age > 60 yr **WITH** multiple cardiac risk factors, systolic BP < 90 mmHg, dyspnea, nonsinus rhythm or new ECG changes suggestive of cardiac ischemia or conduction abnormalities, hematocrit < 30%, or a history of or presence of CHF, CAD, cardiac outflow obstruction, or poor social situation
- ECG: evidence of structural heart disease or conduction disease?
- 2-D echocardiogram if cardiac dysfunction, IHSS, or aortic/mitral stenosis suspected
- Continuous cardiac monitoring to rule out an arrhythmogenic etiology
  - ➤ Positive if symptoms and sinus pause ≥ 2 sec, or sinus bradycardia ≤ 40, or SVT ≥ 180, or type II second-degree AV block, or complete heart block, or sustained VT ≥ 30 sec
- Tilt-table testing: recurrent unexplained syncope with negative cardiac workup
- Stress test to rule out cardiac ischemia for all exertional syncope
- Electrophysiologic test if unexplained syncope **AND** underlying CAD (especially if LVEF < 0.4)
- All cases of cardiac syncope should be reported to the Department of Motor Vehicles

References: J Am Coll Cardiol 2006;47:473; Heart 2007;93:130; Ann Emer Med 2006;47:448; and Ann of Emer Med 2007;49:431.

AORTIC ANEURYSMS

Risk Factors
- Thoracic aortic aneurysm (TAA): Marfan, Turner, or Ehlers-Danlos syndromes; bicuspid AV; HTN; aortitis (Takayasu, giant cell, or syphilitic); and chest trauma
- Abdominal aortic aneurysm (AAA): male sex, age > 65 yr, smoking, HTN, hyperlipidemia, and positive family history (FHx)

Screening
- Abdominal ultrasound for men 65–75 yr with history of smoking or > 60 yr with FHx of AAA

Clinical Presentation
- Asymptomatic; abdominal, chest, or back pain; embolic events distal to aortic aneurysm; or aortic dissection with all associated clinical presentations (see page 39)

Workup
- Screening studies: CXR for TAA and abdominal ultrasound for AAA
- Contrast CT scan of aorta: confirmatory study for both TAA and AAA
- Surveillance studies: for AAA 4–5.4 cm, check an abdominal ultrasound q 6 months
  ➢ TAA, contrast CT scan q 6 months; plus annual echo if moderate–severe AS or AI
- Transthoracic or transesophageal echo: further evaluation of aortic root in TAA
- Preop labs: CBC, chemistry panel, PT, PTT, and ECG; add screening PFTs for smokers
- Screen for CAD, carotid artery disease, and other PAD

Medical Treatment
- Lifestyle changes: smoking cessation; low sodium/cholesterol diet; avoid heavy lifting
- Maintain BP < 120/80 mmHg: ACEI and β-blockers are preferred
- Statins for goals: triglycerides < 150 mg/dL, LDL < 100 mg/dL, and HDL > 40 mg/dL
- Aspirin 81 mg PO daily

Indications for Surgery of Aortic Aneurysms
- AAA: ≥5 cm (women) or ≥5.5 cm (men); symptomatic; or rapidly expanding (>1 cm/yr)
- TAA: ascending ≥ 5.5 cm; descending > 6 cm; growth (>5 mm/yr); AV surgery and > 4 cm

Candidates for Endovascular Repair of Aortic Aneurysms
- Infrarenal AAA +/– iliac aneurysm in high-risk surgical candidates
- Descending TAA starting and ending > 1.5 cm from left subclavian and celiac arteries

Postoperative Medical Management After Aortic Aneurysm Repair
- Perioperative β-blockade titrated to resting heart rate 55–65 bpm
- Maintain SBP in a range 20 mmHg above and below patient's baseline SBP
- Consider continuous epidural anesthesia for postoperative pain control
- Close monitoring for cardiac ischemia, bleeding, and renal dysfunction

References: Circulation 2008;117:1883; 2005;112:1663; 2008;117:2288; 2008;118:188; 2008;117:841; and Curr Opin Crit Care 2006;12:340.

Section 5
Critical Care Medicine

SEVERE SEPSIS AND SEPTIC SHOCK

Definitions
- Severe sepsis is sepsis with sepsis-induced organ dysfunction of at least 1 organ
- Septic shock is severe sepsis with shock refractory to an adequate fluid challenge (~2–3 L)

Sepsis-Induced Organ Dysfunction
- CNS: acutely altered mental status or encephalopathy
- Lungs: acute lung injury (ALI) or adult respiratory distress syndrome (ARDS)
  - ➤ See definitions of ARDS and ALI on pp. 49–50
- Heart: acute myocardial dysfunction (typically LVEF <0.4) or hypotension
- GI: ileus or hepatic dysfunction (total bilirubin >2 mg/dL and liver transaminitis)
- Renal: acute kidney injury
- Hematologic: thrombocytopenia (<100 K), coagulopathy (INR > 1.5 or PTT > 60 sec), or DIC
- Lactic acidosis (lactate >2 mmol/L)

Poor Prognostic Factors in Septic Shock
- APACHE II score ≥25; cirrhosis; chronic cardiopulmonary disease; abdominal compartment syndrome; ARDS; or multi-organ dysfunction syndrome

Management of Severe Sepsis and Septic Shock
- **Early goal-directed therapy (EGDT) endpoints:** recommend a central line and an arterial line
  - ➤ Urine output ≥0.5 mL/kg/hr
  - ➤ Mean arterial pressure (MAP) ≥65 mmHg measured by an arterial line
    - Vasopressors (dopamine or norepinephrine) if MAP < 65 mmHg once adequate CVP (also indicated for life-threatening shock with low CVP until volume resuscitated)
    - Add vasopressin 0.01–0.04 units/min for septic shock refractory to above pressors
  - ➤ CVP 8–12 mmHg (nonintubated) or 12–15 mmHg (intubated or diastolic dysfunction)
  - ➤ Central venous oxygen saturation (ScvO₂ ≥70% or mixed venous O₂ saturation (SvO₂) ≥65%
    - If ScvO₂ <70%, transfuse PRBCs (if necessary) to achieve Hct ≥30%
    - Start dobutamine at 2.5 mcg/kg/min titrated up to 20 mcg/kg/min until ScvO₂ ≥70%
- **Diagnostic studies**
  - ➤ CBCD, chemistry panel, lactic acid, blood cultures × 2, CXR, UA, urine culture, and ABG
  - ➤ Sputum culture if any concerns for pneumonia
  - ➤ Lumbar puncture if unexplained altered mental status or nuchal rigidity
  - ➤ Paracentesis if significant ascites is present
  - ➤ Diagnostic thoracentesis if a moderate–large parapneumonic effusion is present
- **Antibiotic therapy**
  - ➤ Initiate appropriate antibiotics (usually broad spectrum) within 1 hr of organ dysfunction

> Combination therapy advised for neutropenia or if any risk factors for multidrug resistant (MDR) bacteria
>   ○ Risk factors for MDR bacteria: hospitalization for at least 48 hr or prolonged antibiotic use in last 90 d; current hospitalization for >5 d; residence in a long-term care facility; or any healthcare-associated pneumonia.
> De-escalate antibiotics within 48–72 hr once organism isolated and sensitivities known

- **Source control:** accomplish within 6 hr of shock or organ dysfunction
- **Vasopressors**
  > Norepinephrine or dopamine are initial vasopressors (see Table 5-3)
  > Consider adding vasopressin 0.01–0.04 units/min for refractory shock
- **Corticosteroids**
  > Cosyntropin stimulation test is probably of limited utility for patients in septic shock
  > Consider hydrocortisone 200–300 mg/day IV for vasopressor-dependent septic shock
  >   ○ Improves shock reversal at 7 d; no mortality benefit or increase in infections
  > Wean off corticosteroids over 48–72 hr once the patient is off vasopressors
- **Blood product administration**
  > Transfuse packed red blood cells when Hgb <7 g/dL or if needed for EGDT
  >   ○ No role for erythropoietin in sepsis-induced anemia
  > Transfuse platelets when: PLT < 5000/mm³; 5000–30,000/mm³ with bleeding; or <50,000/mm³ and need for surgery or an invasive procedure
- **Mechanical ventilation**
  > Lung-protective ventilation with tidal volume (Vt) 6 mL/kg (predicted body weight)
  > Analgesia and sedation to maintain a calm, comfortable state
  > Keep plateau pressure ≤30 cmH₂O
  > Allow permissive hypercapnia if pH ≥ 7.2 and no increased intracranial pressure
  > Keep head of the bed elevated to 45°
  > Chlorhexidine 15 mL oral rinses bid
  > Daily interruption of continuous sedation and minimize use of benzodiazepines
  > Avoid neuromuscular blockers if possible; less risk of critical illness polyneuropathy
  > Use a weaning protocol with spontaneous breathing trials to assess extubation readiness
  > Use a conservative fluid strategy for patients with ALI or ARDS and who are no longer in shock
- **Glucose control** (no benefit of tight glycemic control between 80–110 mg/dL in medical patients)
  > Insulin drip titrated to keep blood glucose 100–180 mg/dL
- **Renal replacement therapy**
  > Intermittent hemodialysis and continuous venovenous hemofiltration are equivalent
- **Bicarbonate therapy:** consider for severe lactic acidosis with pH < 7.15 (no clear outcome benefit)
- **Deep venous thrombosis prophylaxis**
  > Heparin 5000 units SQ q8h; or LMWH

> Sequential compression devices for all patients
- **Stress ulcer prophylaxis**
  > H_2-blocker, proton pump inhibitor, or sucralfate for patients in septic shock or on a ventilator
- **Nutrition**
  > Start enteral feeds (if possible) once the patient requires no more than low-dose vasopressors
  > Oxepa is the preferred enteral formulation for severe sepsis, septic shock, or ARDS/ALI
- **Drotrecogin-alpha (Xigris)**
  > Indicated for severe sepsis or septic shock with a high risk of death (APACHE II score ≥25 or organ dysfunction of at least 2 organs)
  > For Xigris contraindications, see www.xigris.com/pdf/dosing-guide.pdf
  > Infusion based on actual body weight at 24 mcg/kg/hr × 96 hr
- **Communication with family**
  > Understand what the patient's wishes would be in terms of extent of care.
  > Address spiritual needs and psychosocial concerns.
  > Consider limitation of support or withdrawal of care for patient's failing to improve or for severe deterioration despite maximal medical therapy.

References: Adapted from the 2008 Surviving Sepsis Campaign at Crit Care Med 2008;36:296 *and* NEJM 2001;345:1368; *Chest 2003;124:1016; and Clin Infect Dis 2009;49:93.*

SHOCK

Definition
- A medical condition in which tissue perfusion and oxygen delivery is insufficient for the metabolic demands of the body

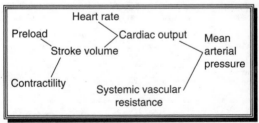

Figure 5-1 Determinants of Blood Pressure and Cardiac Output

Table 5-1 Classification of Shock States

Shock type	PCWP	Cardiac index	SVRI
Cardiogenic (CI < 2.0 L/min)	↑	↓	↑
Hypovolemic	↓	↓	↑
Distributive (sepsis, anaphylactic shock, or spinal shock)	Normal or ↓	Elevated (unless SIRS-related myocardial dysfunction or under-resuscitated patient)	↓
Obstructive (tension PTX, massive PE* or tamponade†)	↑ (tamponade) NL/↑ (PE or PTX)	↓	↑

* Massive PE associated with elevated PA, RA, and CVP pressures, PAD > PCWP, profound hypoxemia, and right heart strain on ECG and echocardiogram.
† Tamponade will show equalization of RA, RV, PAD, and PCWP pressures.
PCWP = pulmonary capillary wedge pressure; SVRI = systemic vascular resistance index; CI = cardiac index; PTX = pneumothorax.

Table 5-2 Treatment of Shock States

Shock	Treatment
Hypovolemic	Aggressive fluid resuscitation
Cardiogenic	Dobutamine; IABP or LVAD; possible revascularization or transplantation
Septic shock	See pp. 45–47
Spinal shock	Judicious fluids; dopamine for bradycardia and hypotension +/− surgical decompression
Anaphylaxis	Fluids; H₁-blocker; H₂-blocker; corticosteroids; epinephrine 1 mg IM
Tamponade	Pericardiocentesis
Tension PTX	Needle decompression 2nd ICS midclavicular line; tube thoracostomy
Massive PE	Support airway and breathing; fluids; thrombolytics and antithrombotics

Table 5-3 Vasopressors

Medication	Dose	Inotropy	Chronotropy	Receptors
Dopamine	≤5 mcg/kg/min	Vasodilation effect		Dopamine rec.
	5–10 mcg/kg/min	Yes	Yes	α = β
	>10 mcg/kg/min	Vasoconstriction effect		α > β
Dobutamine	2.5–20 mcg/kg/min	Yes	Yes	β_1 and β_2 > α_1
		Mild vasodilatation		
Norepinephrine (Levophed)	1–30 mcg/min	Yes	+/−	α > β
Vasopressin (adjunct)	0.01–0.04 U/min	Vasoconstriction Augments catecholamines		V_1/V_2 receptors
Phenylephrine (Neo-Synephrine)	40–180 mcg/min	Vasoconstriction		α_1
Isoproterenol	2–10 mcg/min	Yes	Yes	Pure β-agonist
		Mild vasodilation		

References: Crit Care Med *2005;33:1119*; Crit Care Med *2004;32:691*; JAMA *2005;294:1693*; and N Engl J Med *2001;345:1368*.

HYPERTENSIVE EMERGENCIES

- **Definition:** markedly elevated BP > 220/120 mmHg associated with acute end-organ damage

- Examples: hypertensive encephalopathy (headache, confusion, and papilledema); CHF; acute coronary syndrome; ARF; aortic dissection; ischemic or hemorrhagic stroke; preeclampsia or eclampsia
- Treatment of HTN emergency: cautiously ↓ MAP 25% with IV meds in the ICU × 12–24 hr
- Distinguish from HTN urgency: BP > 180/110 mmHg, but **no end-organ damage**
  ➤ May treat with oral agents and manage with close follow-up as an outpatient

Table 5-4 Management of Hypertensive Emergencies

Medication	IV dosages	Special indications	Cautions
Nitroprusside	0.25–10 mcg/kg/min	CHF or refractory HTN in stroke or aortic dissection; +/– for encephalopathy	Increased ICP; cyanide or thiocyanate toxicity*
Labetalol	20–80 mg IV q 10 min then 0.5–2 mg/min IV	Encephalopathy, ACS[†], aortic dissection, acute stroke, preeclampsia, or pheochromocytoma (pheo)	Bradycardia or heart block; severe bronchospasm; severe CHF
Nitroglycerin	5–200 mcg/min	ACS or CHF	Headache (HA)
Nicardipine	5–15 mg/hour	Acute stroke or preeclampsia	Tachycardia, ACS
Hydralazine	10–20 mg IV q 20 min	Preeclampsia, CHF	Tachycardia, HA
Enalaprilat	0.625–1.25 mg IV q6h	CHF	↓ renal function, ↑ K
Esmolol	500 mcg/kg load then 50–300 mcg/kg/min	ACS[†], aortic dissection, or adjunct for pheo	Bradycardia or heart block
Fenoldopam	0.1–0.3 mcg/kg/min	CHF or ACS or acute kidney injury	Tachycardia or glaucoma

* Risk higher with prolonged use > 24 hr and with severe renal or hepatic impairment.
† Avoid if ACS secondary to cocaine or methamphetamine abuse; treat with nitrates and benzodiazepines.
ACS = acute coronary syndrome; ICP = intracranial pressure; HTN = hypertension.
Adapted from *Chest* 2007;131:1949 and *Circulation* 2008;117:1897.

References: Cochrane Database Syst Rev *2008(1):CD003653* and Chest *2007;131:1949.*

ACUTE RESPIRATORY FAILURE

Acute Hypoxemic Respiratory Failure (severe hypoxia with preserved ventilation)
- Causes: ARDS, pneumonia, CHF, aspiration pneumonitis, pulmonary fibrosis, diffuse interstitial lung disease, pulmonary contusion, PE, pneumothorax, mucous plugging with lung collapse, severe atelectasis, status asthmaticus, or COPD exacerbation

Hypercapnic Respiratory Failure (ventilatory failure with hypoxia)
- Causes: oversedation, brainstem stroke, traumatic brain injury, intracranial hemorrhage, C-spine injury, status asthmaticus, COPD exacerbation, bronchiectasis, obesity-hypoventilation syndrome, severe neuromuscular disorders, myopathies, chest wall disorders, or severe chest trauma
- Ventilatory failure: pH ≤ 7.25; $PaCO_2$ ≥50 mmHg; RR > 35 or RR < 10; and increased work of breathing

Acute Respiratory Distress Syndrome (ARDS)
- ARDS criteria: acute onset; bilateral patchy alveolar infiltrates; PCWP ≤ 18 mmHg (or no clinical evidence for increased left atrial pressure); and PaO_2/FiO_2 ≤ 200

> ARDS facts: 1/3 to 1/2 of pts have a PCWP >18 mmHg; PaO_2/FiO_2 may vary with PEEP
- Acute lung injury (ALI): same criteria as above, except the $PaO_2/FiO_2 = 201$–300
- Etiologies: pneumonia, sepsis, aspiration pneumonitis, shock, drowning, pancreatitis, trauma, pulmonary contusions, inhalation injury, DIC, massive transfusion, or drug overdose
- Treatment
  > Lung-protective ventilation with tidal volumes (Vt) of 6 mL/kg predicted body weight
  > Maintain plateau pressures (Pplat) ≤30 cmH₂O and allow permissive hypercapnia
    ○ Use lower Vt (4–5 mL/kg predicted body weight) if Pplat >30 cmH₂O persistently
  > Conservative fluid strategy preferred if patient is normotensive and nonoliguric
  > Methylprednisolone may be beneficial in **early** ARDS if started within 7 d of diagnosis (ideally within 72 hr): 0.5–2.5 mg/kg/d methylprednisolone as continuous infusion or in divided doses (1 mg/kg/d most commonly used); duration of use unclear
    ○ Decreased ventilator days, ICU length of stay, lung injury scores, multiorgan dysfunction syndrome scores, and a trend toward decreased mortality

References: Lancet 2007;369:1553; NEJM 2006;354:2564; Chest 2007;131:954; Crit Care Med 2008;36:2912; and Crit Care Med 2009;37:1594.

MECHANICAL VENTILATION

Initiating Mechanical Ventilation
Choose the mode of ventilation
- AC if very limited patient effort, heavy sedation, or paralyzed patient (VC or PRVC or PC)
- SIMV if some respiratory effort or patient-ventilator dyssynchrony on AC

Settings for oxygenation
- Initial FiO_2 0.8–1.0; adjust to keep SaO_2 ≥90% or PaO_2 ≥60 mmHg
- Initial PEEP 5 cmH₂O, adjust according to FiO_2 (see PEEP-FiO_2 algorithm in Table 5-5)
- Aim to titrate FiO_2 ≤0.6

Settings for ventilation
- Tidal volume (Vt): 6–8 mL/kg predicted body weight (PBW)
  > PBW for men (kg) = 50 + [2.3 × (height in inches −60)]
  > PBW for women (kg) = 45.5 + [2.3 × (height in inches −60)]
- Ventilator rate: 12–16/min; adjust rate based on $PaCO_2$ and pH
  > Consider initial rate of 20–24/min in acute respiratory distress syndrome (ARDS)
  > Can ↑ rate to 35/min if necessary (watch for auto-PEEP if ↑↑ RR and bronchospasm)
- Keep Pplat ≤30 cmH₂O (decrease Vt for persistently elevated Pplat >30 cmH₂O)

Table 5-5 PEEP-FiO$_2$ Algorithm for Lung Protective Ventilation

FiO$_2$	0.3	0.4	0.4	0.5	0.5	0.6	0.7	0.7	0.7	0.8	0.9	0.9	0.9	1.0	1.0	1.0	1.0
PEEP*	5	5	8	8	10	10	10	10	12	14	14	14	16	18	18	20	22	24

* PEEP measured in cmH$_2$O.
Adapted from ARDS Clinical Trial Network. *NEJM* 2004;351(4):327–336 and *NEMJ* 2000;342(18):1301–1308.

Additional ventilator settings
- I:E ratio: initially 1:2; shorten inspiratory time (It)(i.e., I:E 1:4) for severe bronchospasm; and can prolong It (i.e., I:E 1:1.3) for refractory hypoxia
- Pressure support: if SIMV mode, can adjust between 6–20 cmH$_2$O titrated to patient comfort
- Lung-protective ventilation is indicated for ARDS/acute lung injury or severe sepsis
- Allow permissive hypercapnia (up to PaCO$_2$ ≤80 mmHg) if patient has no increased intracranial pressure or severe right heart disease
- May use sodium bicarbonate drip if necessary to keep pH ≥ 7.2

Monitoring During Mechanical Ventilation
- Continuous cardiac monitor and oximetry
- Ventilator: tidal volume, minute volume, Pplat, and serial arterial blood gases
- End-tidal carbon dioxide (E$_t$CO$_2$) monitors desirable for ventilator weaning

General Guidelines for Mechanical Ventilation
- Adjust ventilation by changing minute volume = tidal volume × respiratory rate
  > Ventilate to pH, **NOT** to PaCO$_2$; allow ↑↑ PaCO$_2$ unless ↑ intracranial pressure (ICP)
- Improving oxygenation: increase FiO$_2$, PEEP, or inspiratory time (if refractory hypoxia)
- Avoid neuromuscular blockers if possible; less risk of critical illness polyneuropathy
- Continuous sedation titrated to patient comfort: sedatives—benzodiazepines or propofol
  > Analgesics: opioids, ketamine (avoid if ↑ ICP), or dexmedetomidine (see Table 5-9)
  > Daily interruption of continuous sedation and assess readiness to extubate daily
- Use an active weaning protocol
- Prophylaxis: head of bed ↑ to 45°, chlorhexidine oral rinses, low-molecular weight heparin or unfractionated heparin, sequential compression devices, and proton pump inhibitor or H$_2$-blocker

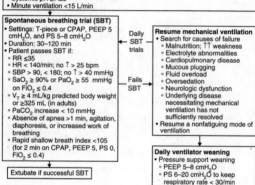

Patient is ready for a spontaneous breathing trial if he/she meets the following criteria:
- Awake, cooperative, and follows commands
- Good gag reflex
- Strong cough
- Minimal secretions
- Hemodynamically stable off vasopressors
- The underlying disease leading to intubation has resolved
- Hemoglobin ≥8 g/dL
- Spontaneous breathing on PEEP < 8
- PaO_2/FiO_2 ratio ≥150–200 (or SaO_2 ≥90% with FiO_2 ≤0.4)
- Systemic pH ≥7.25
- Minute ventilation <15 L/min

Spontaneous breathing trial (SBT)
- Settings: T-piece or CPAP, PEEP 5 cmH_2O, and PS 5–8 cmH_2O
- Duration: 30–120 min
- Patient passes SBT if:
  - RR ≤35
  - HR < 140/min; no ↑ > 25 bpm
  - SBP > 90, < 180; no ↑ > 40 mmHg
  - SaO_2 ≥ 90% or PaO_2 ≥ 55 mmHg on FiO_2 ≤ 0.4
  - V_T ≥ 4 mL/kg predicted body weight or ≥325 mL (in adults)
  - $PaCO_2$ increase < 10 mmHg
  - Absence of apnea >1 min, agitation, diaphoresis, or increased work of breathing
  - Rapid shallow breath index <105 (for 2 min on CPAP, PEEP 5, PS 0, FiO_2 0.4)

Extubate if successful SBT

Daily SBT trials

Fails SBT

Resume mechanical ventilation
- Search for causes of failure
  - Malnutrition; ↑↑ weakness
  - Electrolyte abnormalities
  - Cardiopulmonary disease
  - Mucous plugging
  - Fluid overload
  - Oversedation
  - Neurologic dysfunction
  - Underlying disease necessitating mechanical ventilation has not sufficiently resolved
- Resume a nonfatiguing mode of ventilation

Daily ventilator weaning
- Pressure support weaning
  - PEEP 5–8 cmH_2O
  - PS 6–20 cmH_2O to keep respiratory rate < 30/min
  - Gradually wean PS by 2–4 cmH_2O as tolerated
  - If patient is unable to tolerate PS ventilation, use a backup rate and a comfortable mode of ventilation

FiO_2 = fraction of inspired oxygen; HR = heart rate; $PaCO_2$ = partial pressure arterial carbon dioxide; PaO_2 = partial pressure arterial oxygen; PEEP = positive end-expiratory pressure; PS = pressure support; RR = respiratory rate; SaO_2 = arterial oxygen saturation; SBP = systolic blood pressure; CPAP = continuous positive airway pressure; SIMV = synchronized intermittent mandatory ventilation; V_T = tidal volume. Adapted from *Chest* 2001;120:375S–395S and *Crit Care Med* 2008;36:2753.

Figure 5-2 Weaning and Liberation from Mechanical Ventilators

NONINVASIVE VENTILATION

Potential Indications for Noninvasive Positive Pressure Ventilation (NPPV)
- Moderate–severe COPD exacerbations
- Severe CHF exacerbations

- Acute hypoxemic respiratory failure
- Acute respiratory failure in immunocompromised patients
- Prevention of postextubation respiratory failure in patients with COPD exacerbation

Contraindications for NPPV
- Depressed level of consciousness or severe encephalopathy
- Risk of aspiration or inability to protect airway (poor gag reflex or cough)
- Upper airway obstruction
- Hemodynamic instability or life-threatening arrhythmia
- Recent GI, facial, or oropharyngeal surgery
- Significant upper GI bleed
- Facial deformity, facial trauma, or anatomic abnormality precluding a tight mask application
- Severe claustrophobia

Technique
- Slowly acclimate patient to NPPV
- Initiate BiPAP with iPAP 10 cmH$_2$O/ePAP 4–5 cmH$_2$O
- Increase iPAP titrated to tidal volume (Vt) = 5–7 mg/kg predicted body weight
- Increase ePAP and wean FiO$_2$ to maintain SaO$_2$ ≥90%
- Avoid iPAP ≥25 cmH$_2$O and caution with iPAP >20 cmH$_2$O (causes gastric distension)
- Discourage using a nasogastric tube, which increases the risk of aspiration and mask leak
- Check an ABG after 1–2 hr to assess efficacy

Monitoring Patients on NPPV
- Continuous cardiac monitoring and oximetry
- Observe for decreased work of breathing, agitation, dyspnea, and improved patient comfort
- Monitor for ventilator–patient dyssynchrony and for significant air leaks

Predictors of Failure for NPPV
- Poor cooperation and poor fitting or intolerance of face mask
- Low body mass index ≤23
- Presence of ARDS or Simplified Acute Physiology Score II (SAPS II) score >35
- Initial pH < 7.2 or initial PaCO$_2$ >90 mmHg
- Respiratory process that is unlikely to reverse quickly or that could worsen with time
- Minimal improvement after 1–2 hr of NPPV → consider intubation if code status allows

Table 5-6 Complications of Noninvasive Positive Pressure Ventilation

Minor complications	Major complications
Nasal or sinus congestion	Severe gastric distension
Sinus or ear pain	Pulmonary aspiration
Conjunctival irritation	Pneumothorax
Pressure sore on nasal bridge or cheeks	Pressure ulcers on nasal bridge or face
Mild–moderate gastric distension	Hypotension

References: JAMA 2005;294:3124; Lancet 2006;367:1155; and Crit Care Med 2007;35:2402.

ACUTE INTRACRANIAL HEMORRHAGE

- History/exam
- Onset of symptoms
- GCS score
- CBC, chem. panel, PT, PTT
- Noncontrast head CT scan

For GCS ≤ 8 or increased ICP:
- Intubate → $PaCO_2$ 35 +/– 2 mmHg
- Head of bed elevated to 30–45°
- Isotonic fluids until euvolemic
- Consider mannitol 0.5–1 g/kg IV q4h (if serum osmolality < 310–320 mOsm/L)
- Consider intracranial pressure monitoring
- Sedation and neuromuscular blockade for refractory ICP>20 mmHg

- Maintain normothermia and euvolemia
- Keep glucose < 185 mg/dL
- Sequential compression devices
- H_2-blocker or proton pump inhibitor
- Consider antiepileptic × 7 d for lobar hemorrhages
- Correct coagulopathy with FFP and/or cryoprecipitate
- Platelet transfusion if PLT < 100 K

SAH

Medical mgmt
- Keep MAP < 130 mmHg and SBP < 160 mmHg
  > Labetalol, esmolol, or nicardipine
- Nimodipine 60 mg PO q4h × 21 d

- Cerebral angiogram to locate aneurysm
  > Four-vessel cerebral angiogram
  > Digital subtraction CT angiography
- Surgical clipping or endovascular coiling within 72 hr

ICH

Medical mgmt
- Acute BP management
  > Keep MAP < 130 mmHg or SBP < 180 if preexisting HTN or if suspected/known ↑ ICP
    ○ Labetalol, hydralazine, or nicardipine
  > Keep MAP ≤ 110 mmHg or SBP < 160 if no history of HTN, if postcraniotomy, or NL ICP
- Recombinant FVIIa does not improve survival and is not recommended

Indications for surgical evacuation
- Infratentorial ICH > 3 cm or smaller with neurologic deterioration
- Superficial supratentorial ICH with neurologic deficits
- Young patient with lobar ICH and GCS ≤ 13

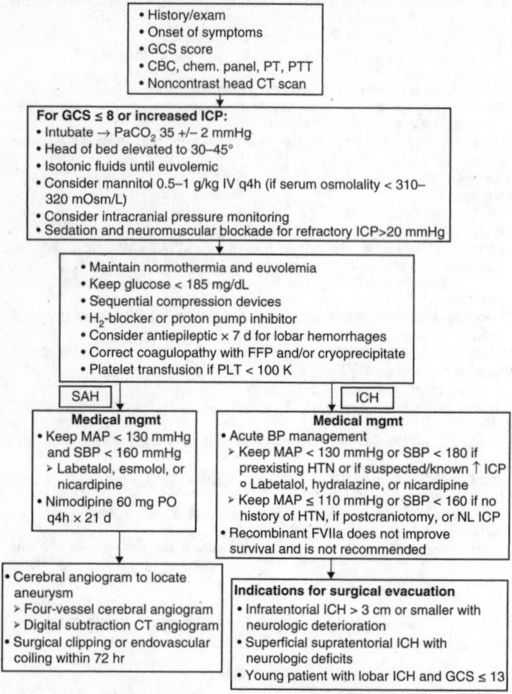

Adapted from *Stroke* 2007;38:2001; *Lancet* 2005;365:387; *Ann Emer Med* 2008;51:S24; *Mayo Clin Proc* 2005;80:420; *Cochrane Database Syst Rev* 2005; Issue 1; and *NEJM* 2008;358:2127.

Figure 5-3 Management of Patients with an Intracranial Hemorrhage

TRAUMATIC BRAIN INJURY (TBI)

Table 5-7 Glasgow Coma Scale

Score	Eye opening	Verbal response	Motor response
6	—	—	Follows commands
5	—	Normal conversation	Localizes pain
4	Spontaneous	Disoriented/inappropriate	Withdraws to pain
3	To voice	Incoherent	Decorticate posturing
2	To pain	Moans	Decerebrate posturing
1	None	None	No movement

Indications for Intubation
- GCS ≤8 or a rapidly declining GCS; hemodynamic instability; respiratory instability; a combative patient precluding the safe completion of studies; or the need for surgery

Indications for Intracranial Pressure (ICP) Monitoring
- GCS ≤8 and either an abnormal CT scan **OR** 2 of following: age >40 yr; motor posturing or focal lateralizing signs; SBP <90 mmHg; or GCS 9–12 and need for a prolonged extracranial operation

General Management Guidelines for TBI
- Positioning: head of bed elevated to 45°, keep neck straight, avoid a tight cervical collar
  - ➤ Recheck the cervical collar after fluid resuscitation, as the neck can swell over time
- DVT prophylaxis: sequential compression devices started immediately
  - ➤ Can add heparin/LMWH once the risk of intracranial bleeding is minimal
- Give seizure prophylaxis with phenytoin or levetiracetam for at least 7 d in severe TBI
- Maintain adequate sedation (e.g., propofol drip) and ventilate to a $PaCO_2 \sim 35$ mmHg
- BP monitoring with an arterial line for severe TBI
- Avoid BP < 90/60 mmHg or PaO_2 <60 mmHg, SaO_2 <90%, fever, pain, anxiety, or coughing
- Expert opinion recommends keeping SBP <160 mmHg for any traumatic intracranial bleed
- Consider early tracheostomy and percutaneous gastrotomy tube during first 7 d for severe TBI
- Nutrition: needs 140% of resting metabolic expenditures if nonparalyzed and 100% of resting metabolic expenditures if paralyzed; ≥15% calories as protein; recommend IMPACT formula
  - ➤ Important to start enteral feeds as early as possible (preferably within the first 24 hr)
- No role for routine antibiotics; or antibiotics during the use of a ventriculostomy drain
- Maintain euvolemia with isotonic fluids; avoid hypotonic fluids.
- No role for steroids, as they may increase mortality in TBI

Management of Increased ICP
- Keep ICP ≤ 20 mmHg and cerebral perfusion pressure ≥60 mmHg (CPP = MAP − ICP)
- Assure proper patient positioning, adequate sedation, no fever, and good ICP waveform

- Hyperosmolar therapy: mannitol 1 g/kg load then 0.25–0.5 g/kg IV q2h prn ↑ ICP if serum osmolality <320 mOsm; or 3% saline at 50 mL/hr to maintain Na ~ 150 mEq/L
- Ventriculostomy with CSF drainage
- Refractory elevated ICP management: consider short-term paralysis; pentobarbital 1 mg/kg/hr; propofol therapy (if blood pressure allows); or decompressive craniectomy
  ➢ Consider a norepinephrine drip to maintain a CPP ≥ 60 mmHg if necessary for ↑↑ ICP

Indications for Surgery for TBI
- Epidural hematoma >30 mL; GCS ≤ 8 with anisocoria; or worsening level of consciousness (LOC) with expanding hematoma
- Acute subdural hematoma with thickness >10 mm or shift >5 mm; ICP > 20 mmHg; GCS decreases ≥2 points between injury and hospital arrival; or depressed LOC with anisocoria
- Intraparenchymal hemorrhage and GCS 6–8 with contusion >50 mL; or frontal/temporal contusions >20 mL and shift >4 mm **OR** cisternal compression
- Posterior fossa bleed/contusion and mass effect or new neurologic defect
- Open depressed skull fracture greater than thickness of skull

Adapted from the 2007 Brain Trauma Foundation Guidelines for the Management of Severe Traumatic Brain Injury, available at www.braintrauma.org.

APPROACH TO THE POISONED PATIENT

General Management of Overdoses
- ABCs; establish vascular access; and continuous cardiopulmonary monitoring
- Empiric treatment of the unresponsive patient
  ➢ Naloxone 0.4 mg IM/IV
  ➢ Thiamine 100 mg IM/IV
  ➢ 1 ampule D_{50} IV
- Intubation for persistent GCS ≤ 8, inability to protect airway, or severe agitation prohibiting necessary testing and evaluation

Workup
- Labs: CBC, chemistry panel, ABG with co-oximetry, serum osmoles, urine drug screen, acetaminophen, salicylate, alcohol +/– lactate levels
- ECG and CXR, and consider head CT scan for any altered mental status

GI Decontamination
- Orogastric lavage for comatose patients with a recent ingestion or for patients with life-threatening ingestions known to be within the last 60 min
- Activated charcoal 0.5–1 g/kg PO/NG indicated for most ingestions in last hour
  ➢ Follow with sorbitol 0.5–1 g/kg PO/NG
  ➢ Ineffective for alcohols, acids, alkali, carbamates, cyanide, DDT, hydrocarbons, iron, lead, lithium, mercury, organophosphates, potassium, and solvents
- Repeated dose of activated charcoal 15–25 g q2–6h considered for: carbamazepine, dapsone, phenobarbital, quinine, and theophylline
- Whole bowel irrigation for enteric-coated/extended-release meds or body packers ("mules")

Ingestions That Benefit from Enhanced Elimination
- **Hemodialysis:** barbiturates, ethanol, ethylene glycol, lithium, methanol, salicylates, and theophylline

- **Hemoperfusion:** carbamazepine, dapsone, methotrexate, phenobarbital, and phenytoin
- **Urine alkalinization:** barbiturates, fluoride, INH, methotrexate, quinolones, and salicylates

Toxidromes

- **Anticholinergic toxidrome:** "red as a beet (flushed), dry as a bone (dry skin), hot as a hare (hyperthermia), blind as a bat (mydriasis), mad as a hatter (delirium), and full as a flask (urinary retention and ileus)" and hypertension, tachycardia, myoclonus, or seizures
  - ➢ **Causes:** amantadine, tricyclic antidepressants, antihistamines, antiparkinsonian meds, low-potency antipsychotics, antispasmodics, atropine, and jimson weed
  - ➢ **Treatment:** activated charcoal; supportive care; and physostigmine 1–2 mg slow IVP
- **Benzodiazepine overdose:** coma, respiratory depression, nystagmus, hypotonia, and hypotension
  - ➢ **Treatment:** supportive care of cardiopulmonary system
- **Cholinergic toxidrome:** SLUDGE (salivation, lacrimation, urination, diarrhea, GI cramps, and emesis) and bradycardia, bronchoconstriction, miosis, and rhinorrhea
  - ➢ **Causes:** carbamate and organophosphate insecticides and cholinesterase inhibitors
  - ➢ **Treatment:** atropine 2 mg IV; or pralidoxime 2 g IV over 30 min then 1 g/hr infusion
- **Opioid overdose:** coma, respiratory depression, miosis, pulmonary edema, ↓ HR/BP
  - ➢ **Treatment:** naloxone 0.1 mg IV q 30 sec cautiously titrated to effect; may need a naloxone infusion of approximately 0.4 mg/hr for overdoses of long-acting opioids
- **Sympathomimetic toxidrome:** tachycardia, hypertension, fever, diaphoresis, mydriasis, hyperreflexia, psychosis, and potentially dysrhythmias or seizures
  - ➢ **Causes:** amphetamines, cocaine, ephedrine, pseudoephedrine, and theophylline
  - ➢ **Treatment:** supportive care; hydration; and benzodiazepines

Management of Acetaminophen Toxicity from ACUTE Ingestions

- Clinical presentation: stage 1—asymptomatic; stage 2—nausea, vomiting, anorexia, RUQ pain, jaundice; stage 3—renal failure, bleeding, ARDS, encephalopathy → coma
- Treatment: N-acetylcysteine 140 mg/kg PO × 1, then 70 mg/kg PO q4h × 17 doses; **OR** 150 mg/kg IV over 60 min, then 50 mg/kg IV over 4 hr, then 100 mg/kg over 16 hr if acetaminophen level within possible or probable hepatotoxicity range in nomogram

Management of Alcohol Intoxications (ethylene glycol, methanol)

- Clinical presentation of alcohols: nausea, confusion, ataxia, slurred speech, sedation, and seizures; severe cases may develop ARDS or cardiac failure
- Ethylene glycol (EG) may cause renal failure, and methanol toxicity causes blindness
- Lab findings: anion-gap acidosis, osmolar gap; ethylene glycol also causes hypocalcemia and urinary calcium oxalate crystals
- Indications for fomepizole or ethanol: serum EG level >20 mg/dL; ingested >100 mL and osmolal gap >10 mOsm/kg; or suspected ingestion and ≥2 of following: pH < 7.3, serum bicarbonate <20 mEq/L, osmolal gap >10 mOsm/kg, or urinary oxalate crystals

Table 5-8 Antidotes for Specific Ingestions

Ingestion or bite	Antidote
Acetaminophen	N-acetylcysteine
Anticholinergics	Physostigmine
Benzodiazepine	Flumazenil (avoid if chronic benzo use)
β-blockers	Atropine, glucagon, and calcium
Wound botulism	Botulism antitoxin
Calcium channel blockers	Atropine, glucagon, and calcium
Carbon monoxide	Supplemental O_2 (hyperbaric in severe cases)
Cholinesterase inhibitors	Atropine; or pralidoxime
Cyanide	Amyl nitrite; sodium nitrite; sodium thiosulfate; and/or hydroxocobalamin; plus 100% oxygen
Digitalis	Digoxin Immune Fab (Digibind)
Ethylene glycol	Ethanol or fomepizole; pyridoxine, thiamine
Heavy metals (arsenic, lead, mercury)	Dimercaprol; EDTA; or penicillamine (copper, lead, and mercury)
Heparin (or LMWH)	Protamine sulfate
Iron	Deferoxamine
Isoniazid	Pyridoxine
Methanol	Ethanol or fomepizole; folinic acid, folate
Methotrexate	Folinic acid
Methemoglobinemia	Methylene blue
Opioids	Naloxone
Organophosphates (and other insecticides)	Atropine or pralidoxime
Snakebites (Crotalids)	Crotalidae Polyvalent Immune Fab
Sulfonylureas	Octreotide, glucagons, and dextrose
Sympathomimetics	Benzodiazepines +/− phentolamine
Thallium	Prussian blue
Warfarin	Vitamin K +/− fresh frozen plasma (if bleeding)

Adapted from *Chest* 2003;123:577.

- Hemodialysis if: worsening vitals; pH < 7.25; refractory renal failure/electrolyte abnormalities

Management of Calcium Channel Blocker Toxicity
- Clinical presentation: altered mental status, fatigue, syncope, hypotension, and bradycardia
- Treatment: fluids and dopamine for hypotension with bradycardia; glucagon 10 mg IVP, then 10 mg/hr for persistent hypotension; calcium chloride 1 g IVP over 10 min, may repeat ×3

Management of Salicylate (ASA) Toxicity
- Clinical presentation: nausea, vomiting → tinnitus, sweating, hyperpnea, delirium → lethargy, respiratory failure, and seizures → cardiac failure and cerebral edema
- Labs: anion-gap acidosis, respiratory alkalosis, hypokalemia, ASA > 20 mg/dL
- Treatment: urinary alkalinization and potassium repletion

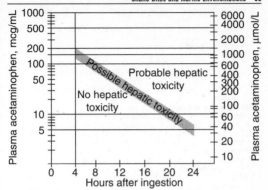

Figure 5-4 Rumack-Matthew Nomogram for Acetaminophen Toxicity from Acute Ingestions

- Hemodialysis if: refractory acidosis or hypotension, seizures, pulmonary edema, rhabdomyolysis, renal failure, ASA level >100 mg/dL or if intubation is needed
- Avoid intubation and mechanical ventilation if possible: increases risk of death

Management of Tricyclic Antidepressant Toxicity

- **Clinical presentation:** anticholinergic toxidrome, sinus tachycardia, drowsiness → delirium, rigidity, prolonged PR/QRS/QT → seizures, hypotension → VF/VT, coma, and respiratory depression
- **Best predictor of seizures or ventricular arrhythmias is a QRS duration >0.16 sec**
  - ➤ Drug levels do not correlate with the degree of cardiac or neurologic toxicity
- **Treatment:** sodium bicarbonate infusion to alkalinize serum to pH 7.45–7.5 for cardiovascular toxicity; isotonic fluids and norepinephrine for hypotension; lorazepam for seizures; and treat arrhythmias with either lidocaine or pacing

References: Clin Med *2008;8:89;* Am Fam Physician *2002;66:807;* Med Letter *2006;4:61;* Emer Med J *2001;18:236;* Emer Med Clin N Amer *2007;25:333; and* Chest *2007;123:577.*

SNAKE BITES AND MARINE ENVENOMATIONS

Snake Bites

- **Clinical presentation:** local tissue injury; extremity swelling; compartment syndrome; rhabdomyolysis; nausea, vomiting; diaphoresis; tingling or numbness
- **Complications:** hypotension; delirium; DIC; paralysis; and acute renal failure
- **Labs:** CBC, chemistry panel, CK, PT, PTT, ECG, UA for blood (myoglobinuria)
- **Treatment:** immobilize affected limb; clean wound; DTaP vaccination; IV fluids for ↓ BP; opioids for pain control; intubation for shock, paralysis, or respiratory failure; mark extent of erythema and follow progression of limb swelling and erythema closely

> Consider fasciotomy for compartment pressures >30 mmHg after antivenom given
> No role for tourniquet, aspiration of venom, excision of the puncture wounds, heparin, steroids, or antifibrinolytic agents
> **Antivenom:** available for crotalids (rattlesnakes, copperheads, and cottonmouths) if <6 hr
> ○ Polyvalent Crotalidae antivenom ovine Fab 4–6 vials IV immediately; repeat q1h until swelling, systemic symptoms, and coagulopathy stable; then give 2 vials IV q6h × 3
> ○ High incidence of serum sickness post-therapy; risk increases with amount infused

Severe Marine Envenomations
- **General management:** ABCs, DTaP vaccination, and good wound debridement
- **Indications for prophylactic antibiotics:** deep extremity wounds; wounds >4 hr from the time of injury; and wounds in immunocompromised hosts
  > Ciprofloxacin or trimethoprim and sulfamethoxazole is usually sufficient
- **Stingrays:** submerse wound in hot water ×30–90 min and copious irrigation of wound
- **Scorpionfish or stonefish:** submerse wound in hot water ×30–90 min, surgical removal of embedded spines, and antivenom for stonefish envenomation
- **Jellyfish:** wash with 5% acetic acid, remove attached tentacles, and use antihistamines
- **Sea urchins:** hot water immersion; remove spines; x-ray area for retained spines

References: Med Clin N Amer 2005;89:1195 and Emer Med Clin N Amer 2004;22:423.

SEROTONIN AND NEUROLEPTIC MALIGNANT SYNDROMES

Serotonin Syndrome (SS)
- **Clinical presentation:** triad of CNS changes (confusion, delirium, agitation, or seizures); neuromuscular dysfunction (hyperreflexia, clonus, shivering, and muscular rigidity); autonomic dysregulation (fever, diaphoresis, hypertension, tachycardia, tachypnea, and mydriasis); nausea/vomiting; diarrhea
  > Spontaneous/inducible clonus of legs > arms > eyes is most important clue for SS diagnosis
  > Develops acutely over 24 hr and usually resolves within 24–48 hr
- Serotonin syndrome typically develops from the combination use of ≥2 serotonergic meds
  > Serotonergic medications: amantadine, amphetamines, bromocriptine, bupropion, buspirone, clomipramine, cocaine, dextromethorphan, dietary supplements (ginseng, St. John's Wort, and tryptophan), doxepin, duloxetine, fenfluramine, granisetron, hallucinogens (LSD and MDMA), imipramine, levodopa, linezolid, lithium, MAO inhibitors, metoclopramide, mirtazapine, nefazodone, ondansetron, opioids (fentanyl, meperidine, pentazocine, and tramadol), ritonavir, SSRIs, sibutramine, trazodone, tricyclic antidepressants, triptans, valproic acid, and venlafaxine
- **Lab findings in severe cases:** metabolic acidosis; ↑ transaminases, CK, and creatinine; +/− DIC
- **Treatment**
  > Discontinuation of offending medications, aggressive hydration, and supportive care

➤ Intubation with neuromuscular paralysis for life-threatening SS (avoid succinylcholine)
➤ Lorazepam 1–2 mg IV q 30 min for agitation, muscle rigidity, myoclonus, and seizures
➤ β-blockers for blood pressure management
➤ Serotonin antagonists: cyproheptadine 12 mg PO × 1 then 4–8 mg PO q4–6h up to 32 mg/d titrated to effect
  ○ Olanzapine 10 mg SL or chlorpromazine 50–100 mg IM added for refractory cases

Neuroleptic Malignant Syndrome
• **Clinical presentation:** high fevers, "lead pipe rigidity," autonomic instability, and AMS
  ➤ Onset over days to weeks, slower resolution than SS, and **no mydriasis or hyperreflexia**
  ➤ Risk factors: dehydration, catatonia, mood disorders, and organic brain syndrome
  ➤ Most common with high-potency antipsychotics (e.g., haloperidol), but can occur with atypical antipsychotics, metoclopramide, promethazine, prochlorperazine, or droperidol
• **Lab findings:** elevated CK, WBC, and liver transaminases; and a metabolic acidosis
• **Treatment**
  ➤ Discontinue offending meds, aggressive hydration, normalize electrolytes and antipyretics
  ➤ Dopamine agonists: bromocriptine 2.5–5 mg PO q8h or amantadine 100–200 mg PO q8h × 10–14 d
  ➤ Dantrolene 2–2.5 mg/kg IV q6h for T ≥ 40°C, coma, respiratory failure, renal failure, or extensive rhabdomyolysis until symptoms controlled, then 1 mg/kg PO q6h × 5–10 d
  ➤ Lorazepam 1–2 mg IV q 30–60 min for autonomic instability, rigidity, and agitation

References: N Engl J Med 2005;352:1112; Crit Care Clin 2008;24:635; and Expert Opin Drug Safety 2008;7:587.

ENVIRONMENTAL EMERGENCIES

Heat Stroke (subtypes are classical versus exertional)
• **Definition:** T > 40°C (104°F) with CNS dysfunction (seizures, delirium, or coma)
• **Risk factors:** age <15 yr or >65 yr; obesity; severe exertion; high environmental heat and humidity; dehydration; alcohol, cocaine, ecstasy, or amphetamine use; meds (pseudoephedrine, ephedrine, phenylpropanolamine, anticholinergics, antihistamines, benzodiazepines, β-blockers, calcium channel blockers, diuretics, laxatives, neuroleptics, phenothiazines, and tricyclic antidepressants)
• **Clinical presentation:** fever, anhydrosis, CNS dysfunction, anorexia, dizziness, headache, nausea, weakness, visual disturbance, distributive shock, DIC, hepatic failure, renal failure, rhabdomyolysis, lactic acidosis, ARDS, and cardiac arrhythmias
• **Labs:** CBC, chemistry panel, CK, urinalysis, urine drug screen, CXR, and ECG
  ➤ Optional labs: ABG, lactic acid, D-dimer, PT, and PTT
• **Treatment**
  ➤ ABCs, remove patient from heat, remove all clothing, IV fluids, and Foley catheter

> External cooling: wet skin, fan, cooling blanket, and ice packs to axilla, groin, neck, and head; or ice water immersion with extremity massage for young patients
> Internal cooling: gastric and bladder cold-water lavage; peritoneal lavage, thoracic lavage, and cardiopulmonary bypass are performed only in extreme cases
> No role for antipyretics, muscle relaxants, benzodiazepines, or dantrolene

Moderate–Severe Hypothermia

- **Definitions:** core temperature 28–32°C (moderate) or <28°C (severe hypothermia)
  > Frostbite: superficial if skin/subcutaneous tissues; deep if bones, joints, or tendons
- **Risk factors:** extremes of age, malnutrition, hypothyroidism, diabetes, adrenal insufficiency, sepsis, environmental temperatures under 0°C, high wind speeds, water immersion, alcohol use, meds (benzodiazepines, meperidine, clonidine, or neuroleptics), immobility; risk of frostbite if wind chill index −20°F or less
- **Clinical presentation:** delirium, amnesia or coma, bradycardia, arrhythmia (e.g., slow Afib), ileus, shock, renal failure, rhabdomyolysis, neuropathy, frostbite, skin blisters, or gangrene
- **Labs:** CBC, chemistry panel, TSH, CK, urine drug screen, PT, PTT, and ABG
  > Other data: CXR, ECG, and urinalysis with microscopic analysis
- **Treatment**
  > ABCs, IV fluids, remove all cold clothing, cardiac monitoring, and a Foley catheter
  > Passive rewarming (mild cases): warming blanket, heat up room, and apply a hat
  > Active rewarming: warm IV fluids and heated oxygen; gastric lavage and bladder lavage with heated fluids in more severe cases
  > Rewarming options for extreme cases with hemodynamic instability: peritoneal lavage, thoracic lavage, heated hemodialysis, or cardiopulmonary bypass
  > Frostbite therapy: place in 40–42°C water ×15–30 min; splint and elevate extremity; keep blisters intact; give DTaP; consider early escharotomy if vascular compromise

Near Drowning

- **Labs:** CBC, chemistry panel, urine drug screen, ECG, CXR, and ABG
- Evaluate patients for head and spinal cord injuries; admit for observation even if asymptomatic
- **Treatment:** ABCs, remove wet clothing, cardiac monitor, IV fluids, Foley catheter, and all passive and active rewarming methods as above if patient is hypothermic
  > Avoid central lines or vasopressor medications, as these can cause arrhythmias
  > Consider early bronchoscopy for foreign body removal and prone ventilation for ARDS
- **Poor prognostic signs:** submersion >5 min, warm water, fresh water, pulseless at scene, ventricular fibrillation, GCS < 8, arterial pH ≤ 7, or initial PaO_2 <60 mmHg

References: Sports Med 2004;34:501; Crit Care 2007;11:R54; Am Fam Physician 2005;71:2133; Can Med Assoc J 2003;168:305; Curr Opin Crit Care 2002;8:578; and BMJ 2003;327:1336.

SEDATION AND PAIN MANAGEMENT IN THE ICU

Table 5-9 Sedation and Analgesia in the ICU

Agent	Half-life/ onset (min)	Intermittent IV dosing	Continuous infusion	Advantages	Disadvantages
Opioids	All opioids hepatically metabolized			**All**	**All**
Fentanyl	1.5-6 hr/ 7-15 min	0.35-1.5 mcg/kg q0.5-1h	0.6-10 mcg/kg/hr	• Analgesia • Sedation • Reversibility **Fentanyl:** rapid onset; short duration and less hypotension	• GI hypomotility • Respiratory depression • Hypotension (especially morphine) **Fentanyl:** chest wall rigidity (rare) **Morphine:** itching
Hydromorphone	2-3 hr/ 10-20 min	10-30 mcg/kg q1-2h	7-15 mcg/kg/hr		
Morphine	3-7 hr/ 10-20 min	0.01-0.15 mg/kg q1-2h	0.07-0.5 mg/kg/hr		
Benzodiazepines	All benzodiazepines hepatically metabolized			**All**	**All**
Diazepam	40-100 hr/ 2-5 min	0.03-0.1 mg/kg q0.5-6h	—	• Anxiolysis • Amnesia • Sedation **Lorazepam:** no prolonged sedation **Midazolam:** rapid onset; preferred for acute agitation	• Respiratory depression • Hypotension possible **Diazepam/midazolam drip:** prolonged sedation **Lorazepam/diazepam drip:** propylene glycol toxicity (acidosis and renal failure)
Lorazepam	8-15 hr/ 5-20 min	0.02-0.06 mg/kg q2-6h	0.01-0.1 mg/kg/hr		
Midazolam	3-11 hr/ 2-5 min	0.02-0.08 mg/kg q0.5-2h	0.04-0.2 mg/kg/hr		
Miscellaneous	Ketamine and dexmedetomidine are hepatically metabolized; propofol is cleared by liver and kidney				
Propofol	26-32 min/ 1-2 min	40 mg q10 min (up to max 2.5 mg/kg)	5-80 (usual) (max 300) mcg/kg/min	Short acting; Easily titratable; Sedation; amnesia	Hypotension; hypertriglyceridemia; rare metabolic acidosis; bradycardia
Ketamine (usually mixed with midazolam in 25:1 ratio)	0.25-2.5 hr/ 1-2 min	1-2 mg/kg IV over 5 min (single dose)	0.1-5 mg/min	Analgesia; amnesia; anxiolysis; ↑ BP; no resp. depression	↑ ICP/ocular pressure/HR; emergence reactions; hypersalivation
Dexmedetomidine	2 hr/ 20-30 min	1 mcg/kg bolus over 10 min	0.2-0.7 mcg/kg/hr (24 h infusion is max duration)	No resp. depression; good for alcohol and drug withdrawal	Hypotension; bradycardia; dry mouth; adrenal suppression; Afib; expensive

Adapted from *Crit Care Med* 2002;30:119; *Crit Care Med* 2006;34:2541; and *Contemp Crit Care* 2007:4:1.

ABSTINENCE SYNDROMES

Table 5-10 Alcohol Abstinence Syndromes

Syndrome	Time from last drink	Clinical presentation
Withdrawal tremulousness	6–36 hr (typically 6–12 hr)	Tremulousness; anxiety; insomnia; headache; palpitations; nausea; anorexia; palpitations
Withdrawal hallucinosis	12–48 hr (typically 12–24 hr)	Visual > auditory or tactile hallucinations; orientation and sensorium usually maintained
Withdrawal seizures	6–48 hr (typically 24–48 hr)	Generalized, tonic-clonic, and typically self-limited
Delirium tremens	48–96 hr (peaks at 120 hr)	Hallucinations; disorientation; sensorium clouded; and marked autonomic instability

Adapted from *Signae Vitae* 2008;3:24 and *Am Fam Physician* 2004;69:1443.

Table 5-11 Clinical Institute Withdrawal Assessment for Alcohol (CIWA-Ar) Scale

Nausea/Emesis	Tremor	Diaphoresis	Anxiety	Agitation
0-None	0-None	0-None	0-None/calm	0-None
1-Mild nausea	1-Can be felt	1-Palms moist	1-Mild anxiety	1-Slight
4-Occasional nausea/dry heaves	4-Moderate tremor	4-Beads of sweat on forehead	4-Moderate anxiety	4-Moderate, fidgety, restless
7-Constant nausea / vomiting	7-Severe tremor	7-Drenching sweats	7-Severe, or panic state	7-Severe, pacing, thrashing about
Tactile disturbance	**Auditory disturbance**	**Visual disturbance**	**Headache or head fullness**	**Level of orientation**
0-None	0-None	0-None	0-None	0-Oriented and can do serial additions
1-Mild itching or paresthesias	1-Very mild sounds	1-Mild sensitivity to light	1-Very mild headache	1-Unsure of date or unable to add
4-Moderate occasional hallucinosis	4-Moderate occasional hallucinosis	4-Moderate occasional hallucinosis	4-Moderate headache	2-Date disorientation by ≤2 d
7-Continuous hallucinosis	7-Continuous hallucinosis	7-Continuous hallucinosis	7-Extremely severe	4-Disoriented to place or person

Score 0–7 for each category except level of orientation where range is 0–4. Minimal withdrawal if score <8 and mild withdrawal if score 8–15; moderate symptoms for score 16–29, severe symptoms for score 30–39, and extremely severe for score ≥40.
Adapted from CIWA-Ar scale in *Brit J Addict* 1989;84:1353.

Table 5-12 Suggested Treatment Regimen for Alcohol Abstinence Syndrome

CIWA-Ar Score*	Intervention†
6–9	Lorazepam 1 mg IV
10–19	Lorazepam 2 mg IV; chlordiazepoxide 25 mg or diazepam 5 mg PO
20–29	Lorazepam 4 mg IV; chlordiazepoxide 50 mg or diazepam 10 mg PO
30–39	Lorazepam 6 mg IV; chlordiazepoxide 100 mg or diazepam 20 mg PO
>40	Lorazepam 8 mg IV q1h until score <30; may need continuous infusion

* Assess CIWA-Ar score q1h × 8 hr if initial score ≥8; then if stable assess q2h × 8 hr; then assess q4h. Assess CIWA-Ar score q4h if initial score <8.

† Consider adjunctive baclofen 10 mg PO tid × 10 d for mild–moderate abstinence syndrome. Consider adjunctive haloperidol 2.5–5 mg IV/IM q2h prn for severe hallucinations, agitation, or combative behavior refractory to benzodiazepines (assure that ≥8 mg lorazepam given in preceding 2 hr). All patients require thiamine 100 mg, folate 1 mg, pyridoxine 100 mg daily, and a multivitamin.

Recommend ICU care for any of the following: CIWA-Ar score ≥35; respiratory distress; hemodynamic instability; unresponsiveness; requires more than 4 mg/hr lorazepam for 3 hr; requires q1h assessment for longer than 8 hr.

Adapted from *J Addict Dis* 2006;25:17; *Pharmacotherapy* 2007;27:510; and *Crit Care Clin* 2008;24:767.

Opioid Abstinence Syndrome
- **Clinical presentation:** flu-like symptoms, mydriasis, lacrimation, rhinorrhea, piloerection, yawning, sneezing, anorexia, nausea, vomiting, and diarrhea
- **Onset (peak/duration):** heroin (36–72 hr/7–10 d); methadone (72–96 hr/14 d)
- **Treatment options**
  - ➤ Opioid agonist: PO methadone 20–35 mg/d or morphine SR 45–120 mg/d; taper over weeks
  - ➤ Nonopioid agents: clonidine 0.1–0.2 mg PO q4h × 3 d then 0.2 mg PO tid and hydroxyzine 25–50 mg PO tid; or lofexidine 0.2 mg PO bid; duration is 10–14 d

Sympathomimetic (Cocaine and Amphetamines) Abstinence Syndrome
- **Clinical presentation:** insomnia, dysphoria, anorexia, nausea, vomiting, fatigue, malaise, restlessness, depression, and craving
- **Onset:** peak symptoms at 48–96 hr and lasts for 7 d
- **Medications for acute withdrawal syndrome**
  - ➤ Propranolol 40–80 mg PO bid for severe withdrawal symptoms; or bromocriptine 2.5–5 mg PO tid for cocaine withdrawal/craving
  - ➤ Consider use of desipramine or bupropion for severe depression
  - ➤ Minimize use of benzodiazepines; but can use if severe restlessness/agitation

References: NEJM *2003;348:1786.*

DIABETIC KETOACIDOSIS

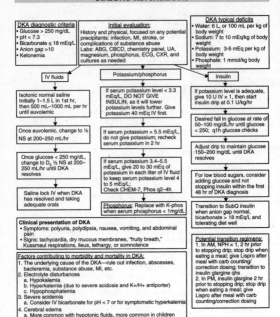

DKA diagnostic criteria
- Glucose ≥ 250 mg/dL
- pH < 7.3
- Bicarbonate ≤ 18 mEq/L
- Anion gap >10
- Ketonemia

Initial evaluation:
History and physical, focused on any potential precipitants: infection, MI, stroke, or complications of substance abuse
Labs: ABG, CBCD, chemistry panel, UA, magnesium, phosphorus, ECG, CXR, and cultures as needed

DKA typical deficits
- Water: 6 L, or 100 mL per kg of body weight
- Sodium: 7 to 10 mEq/kg of body weight
- Potassium: 3-5 mEq per kg of body weight
- Phosphate: 1 mmol/kg body weight

IV fluids

Isotonic normal saline
Initially 1–1.5 L in 1st hr, then 500 mL—1000 mL per hr until euvolemic

Once euvolemic, change to ½ NS at 200–250 mL/hr

Once glucose < 250 mg/dL, change to D5 ½ NS at 200–250 mL/hr until DKA resolves

Saline lock IV when DKA has resolved and taking adequate orals

Potassium/phosphorus

If serum potassium level < 3.3 mEq/L, DO NOT GIVE INSULIN, as it will lower potassium levels further. Give potassium 40 mEq IV first.

If serum potassium > 5.5 mEq/L, do not give potassium; recheck serum potassium in 2 hr

If serum potassium 3.4–5.5 mEq/L, give 20 to 30 mEq of potassium in each liter of IV fluid to keep serum potassium level 4 to 5 mEq/L
Check CHEM-7, Phos q2–4h

Phosphorus: Replace with K-phos when serum phosphorus < 1mg/dL

Insulin

If potassium level is adequate, give 10 U IV x 1, then start insulin drip at 0.1 U/kg/hr

Desired fall in glucose at rate of 50–100 mg/dL/hr until glucose < 250; q1h glucose checks

Adjust drip to maintain glucose 150–200 mg/dL until DKA resolves

For low blood sugars, consider adding glucose and not stopping insulin within the first 48 hr of DKA diagnosis

Transition to SubQ insulin when anion gap normal, bicarbonate > 18 mEq/L and tolerating diet well

Potential transition regimens:
1. In AM, NPH x 1, 2 hr prior to stopping drip; stop drip when eating a meal; give Lispro after meal with carb counting/correction dosing; transition to insulin glargine qhs
2. In PM, insulin glargine 2 hr prior to stopping drip; stop drip when eating a meal; give Lispro after meal with carb counting/correction dosing

Clinical presentation of DKA
- Symptoms: polyuria, polydipsia, nausea, vomiting, and abdominal pain
- Signs: tachycardia, dry mucous membranes, "fruity breath," Kussmaul respirations, ileus, lethargy, or somnolence

Factors contributing to morbidity and mortality in DKA:
1. The underlying cause of the DKA—rule out infection, abscesses, bacteremia, substance abuse, MI, stroke.
2. Electrolyte disturbances
   a. Hypokalemia
   b. Hyperkalemia (due to severe acidosis and K+/H+ antiporter)
   c. Hypophosphatemia
3. Severe acidosis
   a. Consider IV bicarbonate for pH < 7 or for symptomatic hyperkalemia
4. Cerebral edema
   a. More common with hypotonic fluids, more common in children
   b. Beware of obtundation; give mannitol while waiting for your head CT
5. Hypoglycemia (check glucose q1h while on the drip)
6. Return to ketoacidosis: Patients in DKA are ketogenic and remain so for 24–48 hr after their DKA resolves. Should patients become hypoglycemic, give them more sugar. DON'T stop their insulin completely if possible.

Adapted with permission from Mark Lepore, MD. Information from *Postgrad Med J* 2007;83:79; *Diab Care* 2003;26:S109; *Endocrinol Metab Clin N Am* 2006;35:725; *Am Fam Physician* 1999;60:456–457 and *Diab Care* 2006;29:2739.

Figure 5-5 Management of Diabetic Ketoacidosis (DKA)

HYPERGLYCEMIC HYPEROSMOLAR STATE

Diagnostic criteria: serum glucose >600 mg/dL; pH > 7.3; bicarbonate >15 mg/dL; serum osmolality (sOsm) >320 mOsm/kg; and no more than small serum ketones

Clinical features: lethargy, weakness, tachycardia, polyuria, polydipsia, altered mental status, and possibly focal seizures

Initial labs: elevated BUN/crt; increased serum osmolality; and pseudo-hyponatremia

Workup: CBCD, chemistry panel, ABG, ECG, CXR, sOsm, UA, blood and urine cultures

Lab monitoring: chemsticks every hour; and CHEM-7, phosphate, and sOsm every 2–4 hr

Precipitants: same precipitants as DKA plus dehydration, renal failure, and poor access to fluids

Treatment

- Search for and treat the precipitating cause
- Fluids: administer 1–1.5 L NS in 1st hr; follow with 500–1000 mL/hr NS until euvolemic
  - ➤ Typical volume depletion is 8–10 liters
  - ➤ Once euvolemic, ongoing fluids will depend on the corrected SNa and the sOsm
    - ○ If sOsm <320, give 500 mL/hr NS × 2 hr then 250 mL/hr 0.45% NS
    - ○ If sOsm >320 and ↑ corrected SNa, give 0.45% NS 500 mL/hr × 2–4 hr then 250 mL/hr
  - ➤ Once glucose <300 mg/dL, change fluids to D$_5$ ½ NS at 200–250 mL/hr
- Insulin: give insulin 0.1 units/kg (or 5 units) IVP then start an insulin drip at 0.05 units/kg/hr
  - ➤ Always restore volume before giving insulin; otherwise, severe hypotension can occur
  - ➤ If initial serum K < 3–3.5 mEq/L, give 40 mEq KCl prior to administering insulin
  - ➤ Desire ↓ glucose 50–100 mg/dL/hr; and ↓ sOsm 3 mOsm/kg/hr until glucose <300 mg/dL
  - ➤ Transition to SQ insulin or oral diabetic agents once sOsm <320, glucose <300, and patient eating
- Electrolytes
  - ➤ Add 20–40 mEq/L potassium to IVF once serum K < 5 mEq/L and urine output adequate
  - ➤ Replete phosphate with KPhos once serum phosphate <1 mg/dL

References: Postgrad Med J *2007;83:79;* Diab Care *2003;26:S109; and* Endocrinol Metab Clin N Am *2006;35:725.*

VENTILATOR-ASSOCIATED PNEUMONIAS

Table 5-13 Risk Factors for MDR Bacteria Causing Nosocomial Pneumonia

Presence of risk factors for HCAP
• Hospitalized >48 hr in last 90 d
• Resident of a long-term care facility
• Home wound care or infusion therapy
• Chronic hemodialysis in last 30 d
• Attended hospital clinic in last 30 d
• Family member with a MDR organism
• Antimicrobial therapy in last 90 d
• Current hospitalization for ≥5 d
• Immunocompromised state
• High incidence of drug-resistant bacteria in the community or hospital

MDR = multidrug resistant.
Adapted from *Amer J Resp Crit Care Med* 2005;171:388.

Antibiotic Strategies for Ventilator-Associated Pneumonias
• Start broad-spectrum antibiotics and de-escalate to organism-specific therapy within 48–72 hr
• β-lactams infused over 3 hr, and fluoroquinolones are administered in high doses
• Once-daily aminoglycosides are more effective than q8h dosing
• Duration: immunocompetent, non-neutropenic patients with good clinical response; 7–8 d
  ➢ Consider 15-d course for nonfermenting GNRs (e.g., Pseudomonas aeruginosa)
    ○ May be safe to use monotherapy after 5–7 d once susceptibilities are known

Prevention of Ventilator-Associated Pneumonias
• Use noninvasive positive pressure ventilation when possible for acute respiratory failure; daily assessment of readiness to extubate; keep head of bed ≥45°; avoid unnecessary ventilator circuit changes; good hand hygiene; chlorhexidine oral rinses bid; acid suppression therapy; selective gut decontamination with polymixin, aminoglycosides, and amphotericin B for ventilated trauma patients; and possible benefit from continuous suctioning of subglottic secretions

References: Amer J Resp Crit Care Med *2005;171:388;* Clin Infect Dis *2008;46:S296;* Amer J Inf Cont *2006;34:84;* Crit Care Med *2008;36:994; and* Ann Pharmacother *2007; 41:235.*

Suspected ventilator-associated pneumonia
- Mechanical ventilation for at least 48 hr
- CXR with new or progressive pulmonary infiltrate
- Temperature > 38°C (100.4°F) or < 36°C (96.8°F)
- Purulent sputum
- Serum WBC > 10,000 or < 4000 cells/mm^3
- $PaO_2/FiO_2 \leq 240$ in absence of ARDS

Workup: blood culture × 2; culture and Gram stain of lower respiratory tract (endotracheal aspirate, bronchoalveolar lavage, or protected specimen brush sample)

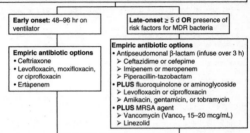

Early onset: 48–96 hr on ventilator

Empiric antibiotic options
- Ceftriaxone
- Levofloxacin, moxifloxacin, or ciprofloxacin
- Ertapenem

Late-onset ≥ 5 d OR presence of risk factors for MDR bacteria

Empiric antibiotic options
- Antipseudomonal β-lactam (infuse over 3 h)
  ➤ Ceftazidime or cefepime
  ➤ Imipenem or meropenem
  ➤ Piperacillin-tazobactam
- **PLUS** fluoroquinolone or aminoglycoside
  ➤ Levofloxacin or ciprofloxacin
  ➤ Amikacin, gentamicin, or tobramycin
- **PLUS** MRSA agent
  ➤ Vancomycin (Vanco$_T$ 15–20 mcg/mL)
  ➤ Linezolid

- De-escalate antibiotics based on culture results within 48–72 hr
- If clinically improved, cultures negative, and CPIS* ≤ 6 at 72 hr, consider discontinuing antibiotics
- If cultures negative and clinical worsening at 72 hr, search for other pathogens or sites of infection, or consider noninfectious disease processes

Duration of treatment
- VAP in immunocompetent, non-neutropenic pts with good clinical response: 7–8 d
- VAP from nonfermenting, gram-negative rods: pseudomonas, acinetobacter, flavobacterium, *Burkholderia cepacia*, *Burkholderia pseudomallei*, and *Stenotrophomonas maltophilia*: 15 days; unclear if ongoing dual therapy superior to monotherapy once susceptibilities are known (may be safe to switch to monotherapy after 5–7 d)

* CPIS = Clinical Pulmonary Infection Score available at http://ajrccm.atsjournals.org/cgi/reprint/168/2/173.
Adapted from *Amer J Resp Crit Care Med* 2005;171:388; *CID* 2008;46:S296; and *Ann Pharmacother* 2007;41:235.

Figure 5-6 Management of Suspected Ventilator-Associated Pneumonia

BRAIN DEATH DETERMINATION

Definition: irreversible loss of brain function, including brainstem function
Causes of acute CNS catastrophe: head injury, intracranial bleed, hypoxic-ischemic brain injury, massive ischemic strokes, fulminant hepatic failure, or severe meningoencephalitis
Clinical criteria for brain death declaration:
- Core temperature >95°F
- No effect of CNS-depressant drugs/meds or neuromuscular blocking agents
- Absence of any confounding metabolic or endocrine disorders
- Absence of cranial nerve function
  > Absence of the following reflexes: pupillary light, corneal, oculocephalic (doll's eyes), oculovestibular (cold caloric testing), sucking, rooting, and gag reflexes
  > No swallowing, yawning, blinking, grimacing, or coughing
- No motor response to noxious stimulation, excluding spinal reflexes
- Absence of spontaneous respirations as determined by an apnea test

Apnea Testing
- Preoxygenate patient with 100% FiO_2 for 20 min
- Start test with $PaCO_2$ ~40 mmHg and pH 7.35–7.45
- Disconnect ventilator and administer oxygen by tracheal cannula at 8–10 L/min
- Maintain SBP ≥90 mmHg during entire test (may use vasopressors if necessary)
- Observe for any spontaneous respirations
- Draw an ABG after 8–10 min and reconnect ventilator
- Positive test if $PaCO_2$ ≥60 or ↑ > 20 mmHg, pH ≤ 7.3, and no spontaneous respirations noted

Alternative Methods to Confirm Brain Death
- Electroencephalogram reveals no electrocerebral activity for at least 30 min
- Cerebral scintigraphy study or cerebral angiogram demonstrates no cerebral blood flow
- Transcranial Doppler ultrasonography with absence of diastolic or reverberating flow

Organ Donation
- Always contact local organ procurement agency to discuss options with family.
References: NEJM 2001;344:1215 and Neurology 1995;45:1012.

EVALUATION OF THE COMATOSE PATIENT

Etiologies of Coma
- Traumatic brain injury; intracranial hemorrhage; hypoxic-ischemic encephalopathy; brain tumor; cerebral vein thrombosis; meningoencephalitis; brain abscess; status epilepticus; hypertensive encephalopathy; massive ischemic stroke; brainstem disorder; osmotic demyelination syndrome; toxic ingestion; carbon monoxide poisoning; severe hypoglycemia; diabetic ketoacidosis; hyperglycemic hyperosmolar coma; severe hyponatremia/hypernatremia or hypercalcemia; Wernicke encephalopathy; adrenal crisis; myxedema coma; or panhypopituitarism

Table 5-14 Disorders of Consciousness

Disorder	Arousal* (state of wakefulness)	Awareness	Sleep/wake cyclic patterns	Motor function	Respiratory function	EEG activity	Cerebral metabolism (% activity)
Brain death	Absent	Absent	Absent	None	Absent	Electrographic silence	0%
Coma (GCS ≤8)	Absent	Absent	Absent	Nonpurposeful	Variable†	Polymorphic delta or theta	<50%
Vegetative state	Present	Absent	Present	Nonpurposeful	Present	Polymorphic delta or theta; sometimes slow alpha	40–60%
Minimally conscious state	Present	Partial	Present	Intermittently purposeful	Present	Mixed theta and alpha	50–60%
Akinetic mutism	Present	Partial	Present	Paucity of movement	Present	Diffuse nonspecific slowing	40–80%

*Comatose patients have no eye opening.
†Disordered breathing patterns common in coma, Cheyne-Stokes respiration, central hyperventilation syndrome, apneustic breathing, or ataxic breathing.
Adapted from *Crit Care Med* 2006;34:31.

- Bag-valve mask ventilation with 100% FiO_2
- Establish vascular access; check chemstick
- Give "coma cocktail"
  - ➢ Thiamine 100 mg IV
  - ➢ 50 mL D_{50} (25 g glucose) IV (if glucose < 60 mg/dL)
  - ➢ Naloxone 0.4–2 mg IV (can repeat q 3 min if effective)
  - ➢ Flumazenil 0.2 mg IV q 1–2 min (max 1 mg) **only if benzodiazepine OD and no history of chronic benzodiazepine use or alcohol abuse**
- Perform a quick neurologic exam prior to paralyzing patient

- Intubate if GCS ≤ 8
- Ventilate to normal pH; keep SaO_2 ≥ 92%
- Maintain a MAP > 70 mmHg
- If ↑ ICP, keep $PaCO_2$ ~ 35 mmHg; give mannitol 0.5–1 g/kg IV; place ICP monitor

- **Labs**: CBCD, chem panel, ABG, TSH, ECG, CXR, cardiac enzymes, serum osmoles, urine drug screen, acetaminophen, salicylate and blood alcohol levels, urinalysis, and blood cultures × 2 (if infection possible)
- For overdoses: gastric lavage for ingestions ≤ 1 hr; then activated charcoal
- Noncontrast head CT

- Consider an EEG and lumbar puncture if etiology remains unclear
- Brain MRI unlikely to alter management but could be considered in equivocal cases

Adapted from *Crit Care Med* 2006;34:31.

Figure 5-7 Approach to the Comatose Patient

Section 6
Perioperative Care and Consultative Medicine

PERIOPERATIVE CARDIOVASCULAR EVALUATION AND MANAGEMENT

Number of risk factors	Revised Cardiac Risk Index	Rate of cardiac complications*
0	I	0.4–0.5%
1	II	0.9–1.3%
2	III	4–6.6%
3–4	IV	9.2–18%
5	V	32%

- Emergency surgery → directly to the OR
- **Presence of any major clinical risk predictors**: ACS,[†] decompensated CHF, arrhythmias[‡] or severe aortic or mitral stenosis? → **Delay/cancel surgery or coronary angiogram**
Revised Cardiac Risk Index
Risk factors: ischemic heart disease[∥]; history of CHF[§]; history of CVA/TIA; diabetes mellitus; creatinine > 2 mg/dL.

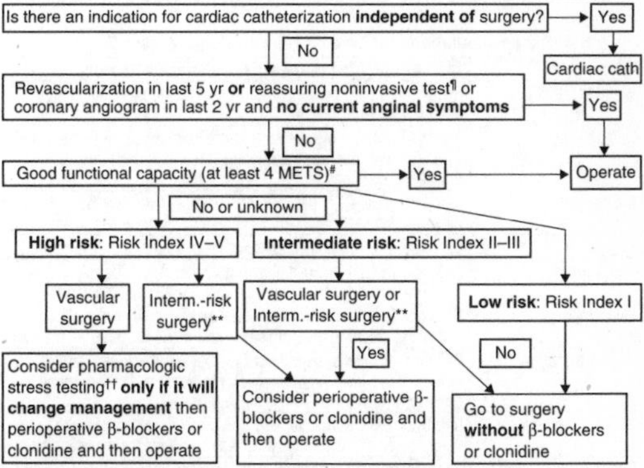

Is there an indication for cardiac catheterization **independent of** surgery? → Yes → Cardiac cath

No

Revascularization in last 5 yr **or** reassuring noninvasive test[¶] or coronary angiogram in last 2 yr **and no current anginal symptoms** → Yes

No

Good functional capacity (at least 4 METS)[#] → Yes → Operate

No or unknown

High risk: Risk Index IV–V   **Intermediate risk**: Risk Index II–III

Vascular surgery | Interm.-risk surgery** | Vascular surgery or Interm.-risk surgery** | **Low risk**: Risk Index I

Consider pharmacologic stress testing[††] **only if it will change management** then perioperative β-blockers or clonidine and then operate

Yes → Consider perioperative β-blockers or clonidine and then operate

No → Go to surgery **without** β-blockers or clonidine

* Combined endpoint of MI, CHF, ventricular fibrillation, complete heart block, or cardiac arrest.
† Post-MI angina, unstable angina, recent NSTEMI, or NYHA class III/IV angina.
‡ High-grade atrioventricular block, symptomatic ventricular arrhythmias with heart disease, supraventricular arrhythmias with a rapid ventricular rate, or symptomatic bradycardia.
§ History of CHF, paroxysmal nocturnal dyspnea, pulmonary rales, S_3 gallop, or consistent CXR.
∥ History of MI, prior CABG or PCI or positive exercise stress test, current angina or nitrate use for chest pain or an ECG with pathologic Q waves.
¶ Positive: ≥10–15% cardiac ischemia or ≥5 segments abnormal on dobutamine stress echo. Negative: <10–15% cardiac ischemia or 0–4 segments abnormal on dobutamine stress echo.
# <4 METs (metabolic equiv.): walking 1–2 blocks, light housework, or with activities of daily living; 4 METs: climb flight of stairs, heavy house work, bowling, dancing, golf, or doubles tennis.
** Vascular surgery, intraperitoneal, carotid endarterectomy, or head/neck, orthopedic, or prostate surgery.
†† Adenosine if unable to exercise and no asthma/COPD, dobutamine if unable to exercise and asthma/COPD, cardiolyte test if >250 pounds and thallium test if <250 pounds.
Adapted from *Circulation* 1999;100:1043; *J Am Coll Cardiol* 2002;39:542; and *J Am Coll Cardiol* 2007;50:159.

Figure 6-1 Perioperative Cardiovascular Evaluation

- No role for prophylactic coronary revascularization prior to major noncardiac surgery even if Revised Cardiac Index class IV–V (CARP study)
- Indications for preoperative coronary artery bypass grafting or percutaneous coronary intervention are identical to the standard indications for these procedures

Indications for Medications to Prevent Perioperative Cardiac Events
- Perioperative β-blockers
  > Indicated for patients with an intermediate–high clinical risk (Revised Cardiac Risk II–V) undergoing vascular or intermediate-risk surgery (see Table 6-1)
  > May start β-blockers immediately prior to surgery and continue 1 wk postop
  > Titrate β-blockers to resting heart rate 55–65 (decreases periop CV events 80%)
  > Contraindications to β-blockers: decompensated CHF, 2° or 3° atrioventricular block, hypotension, severe bronchospasm or symptomatic bradycardia <50 bpm
- Perioperative clonidine 0.2 mg PO × 1 and 0.2-mg patch applied the night before surgery; then 0.2 mg PO × 1 the morning of surgery; remove patch in 4 d; use if β-blockers contraindicated
- Perioperative statin use before major vascular surgery may decrease death or MI

Table 6-1 Recommendations for Testing Prior to Nonemergent Surgery

Test	Indications for preoperative laboratory Testing
White blood count	Symptoms to suggest infection, myeloproliferative disorder, or use of myelotoxic drugs
Hemoglobin	Anticipated large blood loss, symptoms/history of anemia, renal disease, liver disease, hematologic disorders, bleeding diathesis, extremes of age, anticoagulant use
Electrolytes	Renal disease, CHF, DM, adrenal disease, liver disease, hypertension, and meds that can affect electrolytes
Glucose	Diabetes, metabolic syndrome, or morbid obesity
Renal panel	Age >50 yr, HTN, heart disease, diabetes, liver disease, malnutrition, major surgery, and meds that can affect kidneys
Liver panel	Chronically ill, malnourished, liver disease, major surgery, endocrine disease, renal disease, and meds that can affect liver
PT/PTT/platelet	Bleeding diathesis, liver disease, myeloproliferative disorder, malnutrition, anticoagulant use, recent antibiotic use, renal disease, and planned major surgery
ECG	DM, CKD, CAD, PVD, CVA, CHF, AAA, carotid artery disease, unexplained chest pain or dyspnea, or planned major surgery
Chest x-ray	Age >50 yr, known cardiac or pulmonary disease, active cardiac or pulmonary symptoms, abnormal lung exam or morbid obesity
2-D echocardiogram	Unexplained dyspnea, clinical signs of heart failure or history of CHF with worsening dyspnea, or deterioration in clinical status
Urinalysis	Urinary tract symptoms or genitourinary procedure
Urine pregnancy test	Any woman of childbearing age undergoing surgery

PT = prothrombin time; PTT = partial thromboplastin time; PLT = platelets; ECG = electrocardiogram; DM = diabetes; CKD = chronic kidney disease; CAD = coronary artery disease; PVD = peripheral vascular disease; CVA = cerebrovascular accident; AAA = abdominal aortic aneurysm; HTN = hypertension. Adapted from *Anesthesiology* 2002;96:485–496; *Med Clin N Amer* 2003;87:7–40; and *J Am Coll Cardiol* 2007;50:e159.

Recommended Wait Times Prior to Elective or Nonurgent Operations
- Post-MI (4–6 wk); postangioplasty (2 wk); post-bare metal stent placement (30 d); post–drug-eluting stent placement (12 mo); post-stroke (8 wk)

Postoperative Monitoring
- Patients at high clinical risk should have cardiac monitoring for 24–48 hr after major noncardiac surgery
- ECG immediately postop and daily × 2 d and troponin I daily × 2 d

References: J Am Coll Cardiol *2003;42:234;* Chest *2008;133;71, 381;* Circulation *2002; 105;1257;* Arch Intern Med *2004;164:1729;* J Am Coll Cardiol, *2006;47:2343;* J Am Coll Cardiol *2007;50:1707; and* J Vasc Surg *2004;39:967.*

PERIOPERATIVE PULMONARY EVALUATION AND MANAGEMENT

Preoperative Risk Stratification
- Few patients have an absolute pulmonary contraindication to surgery
- Indications for an arterial blood gas: resting hypoxia; risk for chronic hypercapnia; or anticipated lung resection surgery

Table 6-2 Risk Factors for Perioperative Pulmonary Complications*

• Age >60 yr	• COPD
• Smoking within 8 wk of surgery	• CHF
• Poor general health (ASA ≥3)†	• Elevated arterial CO₂ pressure
• Emergency surgery	($PaCO_2$ ≥45 mmHg)
• Thoracic, abdominal aortic aneurysm, neurosurgery, head and neck or upper abdominal surgery	• Functional dependence for ADLs
	• Impaired sensorium
• Surgery lasting >3 hr	• Malnourished (albumin <3.5 g/dL)
• General anesthesia	• Renal failure (blood urea nitrogen [BUN] ≥21 mg/dL)
• Long-acting neuromuscular blockade	• Transfusion >4 U of blood

Obesity alone or asthma does not appear to increase risk. ADL = activities of daily living.
* Perioperative pulmonary complications include atelectasis, pneumonia, or respiratory failure.
† American Society of Anesthesiologists Classification at www.asahq.org/clinical/physicalstatus.htm.
Adapted from *Ann Intern Med* 2006;144:575.

Table 6-3 Postoperative Respiratory Failure Index

Factor	Score	Factor	Score
Type of surgery		Albumin <3 g/dL	9
AAA repair	27	BUN >30 mg/dL	8
Thoracic surgery	21	History of COPD	6
Neurosurgery, upper abdomen, or peripheral vascular surgery	14	Partially or fully dependent functional status	7
Neck surgery	11	Age ≥70 yr	6
Emergency surgery	11	Age 60–69 yr	4

Class	Points	Incidence of postoperative respiratory failure
1	≤10	0.5%
2	11–19	1.8%
3	20–27	4.2%
4	28–40	10.1%
5	>40	26.6%

Adapted from *Ann Intern Med* 2006;144:575.

- Preoperative spirometry should **not** be used to prevent surgery but rather as a tool to optimize preoperative lung function. Appropriate if the patient:
  - ➢ Has asthma or COPD and airflow obstruction that has not been optimized
  - ➢ Has unexplained dyspnea or cough and will undergo major surgery
  - ➢ Will be undergoing lung resection surgery—requires FEV_1 >60% predicted

Interventions to Reduce Perioperative Risk

- Smoking cessation: beneficial if patient quits ≥8 weeks prior to surgery
- Inhaled tiotropium 1 puff daily for COPD +/– β_2-agonists for wheezing
- Oral or inhaled steroids and inhaled tiotropium if COPD or asthma and pulmonary function not optimal (no increased risk of infections, but potential for adrenal suppression if ≥20 mg/d prednisone for ≥3 weeks)
- Defer elective surgery for acute exacerbations of pulmonary disease
- Consider shorter procedures (<3 hr), laparoscopic approach, and spinal/epidural or regional anesthesia rather than general anesthesia for high-risk patients
- Avoid long-acting neuromuscular blockers (e.g., pancuronium)
- Postoperative lung expansion maneuvers and early mobilization recommended
- Consider postoperative epidural analgesia for thoracic or upper abdominal surgery

References: Ann Intern Med 2006;144:575; Anesth Clin N Am 2004;22:77; and Ann Surg 2000;232:242.

PERIOPERATIVE MANAGEMENT OF ANTICOAGULATION AND ANTITHROMBOTICS

Table 6-4 Perioperative Anticoagulation Based on Risk of Thromboembolism

Perioperative risk of thromboembolic event	Conditions	Management
Low (<5%/yr)	• Nonvalvular Afib with CHADS$_2$ score* ≤3 • St. Jude valve—aortic position • VTE >90 d ago • Nonrecurrent stroke/TIA	• Stop warfarin 5 d prior to surgery • Proceed with surgery if INR <1.5 on day of surgery
Intermediate (5–10%/yr)	• VTE 30–90 d ago • History of ≥2 strokes/TIAs • St. Jude valve—mitral position • Older mechanical aortic valve	• Stop warfarin 5 d prior to surgery • Start enoxaparin† 1 mg/kg SQ q12h 36 hr after last warfarin dose
High (>10%/yr)	• VTE in last month • Valvular Afib • Cardioembolism from Afib or a mechanical heart valve • Hypercoagulable state • Acute intracardiac thrombus • Older mechanical mitral valve	• Stop enoxaparin 24 hr preop • Restart enoxaparin 1 mg/kg SQ q12h on postop day 1 • Overlap enoxaparin and warfarin ≥5 d and until INR 2–3 × 24hr

VTE = venous thromboembolism

* See Table 4-12.

† Use unfractionated heparin for wt >155 kg; dose adjust for CrCl 15–30, and avoid if CrCl <15 mL/min.

Adapted from Clev Clin J Med 2005;72:157.

Table 6-5 Regimens for DVT Prophylaxis in Medical and Surgical Patients

Category	Options for DVT prophylaxis
Low-risk patients • Age <40 yr, minor surgery*, no risk factors (RFs)[†]	• Early ambulation • Leg exercises
Moderate-risk patients • Minor surgery + RFs[†] • Surgery in pts 40–60 yr • Major surgery[¶] + no RFs[†]	• Heparin[‡] 5000 U SQ q8h started 2h preop • LMWH[§] • Fondaparinux[∥] 2.5 mg SQ daily • GCS or IPC
High-risk patients • Surgery, 40–60 yr + RFs[†] • Surgery > 60 yr • Major surgery[¶] < 40 yr + RFs[†] • High-risk medical patient[†]	• Heparin[‡] 5000 U SQ q8h started 2 hr preop • LMWH[§] • Fondaparinux[∥] 2.5 mg SQ daily • GCS or IPC
Highest-risk patients • Major surgery[¶] > 40 yr + RFs[†] • THA, TKA, or HFS • Major trauma[#] • Spinal cord injury[#] • Critically ill medical patient	IPC **PLUS** one of the following: • Heparin[‡] 5000 U SQ q8h started 2 hr preop • LMWH[§] • Fondaparinux[∥] 2.5 mg SQ daily • Warfarin titrated to INR 2–3 option for THA or TKA
Moderate- to high-risk patients at high risk for bleeding	• GCS or IPC until bleeding risk is low • Initiate thromboprophylaxis when bleeding risk low

RF = risk factor; GCS = graduated compression stockings; IPC = intermittent pneumatic compression devices; THA = total hip arthroplasty; TKA = total knee arthroplasty; HFS = hip fracture surgery; CA = cancer.

*Eye, ear, dermatologic, laparascopic, or arthroscopic operations.

† Severe burns, immobility, prior VTE, active cancer, stroke with paresis, inherited thrombophilia, polycythemia, myeloproliferative disorder, obesity (BMI >30), CHF, nephrotic syndrome, inflammatory bowel disease, acute MI, acute respiratory failure, sickle cell disease, paroxysmal nocturnal hemoglobinuria, pregnancy, recent trauma, central venous catheter, mechanical ventilation, severe sepsis, shock, and use of the following meds: tamoxifen, raloxifene, thalidomide, lenalidomide, darbepoetin, epoetin alfa, bevacizumab, hormone replacement therapy, or systemic chemotherapy.

‡ Caution starting heparin if initial PLT <50K, and discontinue if PLT count falls ≥50% or to <100K.

§ LMWH = low molecular weight heparins: enoxaparin 40 mg SQ daily starting 1–2 hr preop or 30 mg SQ q12h starting 12–24 hr postop; dalteparin 2500 U SQ starting 1–2 hr preop and 6–8 hr postop, then 5000 U SQ daily (not approved for TKR); tinzaparin 75 U/kg SQ daily starting 10–12 hr before THR/TKR; dosage adjustment required for CrCl 15–30 mL/min and adjust dose based on anti-FactorXa levels if weight > 155 kg; avoid if CrCl <15 mL/min; caution if initial platelet <50K, and discontinue if platelets fall ≥50% or to a level <100K.

∥ Give 6–8 hr postop; avoid if CrCl <30 mL/min, weight <50 kg, thrombocytopenia with positive antiplatelet antibodies, epidural infusions, or endocarditis; no antidote if active bleeding develops; T$_{1/2}$ ~ 18 hr.

¶ Thoracic, intraperitoneal, bariatric, open urologic and gyn, cardiac, neurosurgical, and cancer operations.

Thromboprophylaxis can generally be started within 36 hr of major trauma or spinal cord injury unless intracranial bleeding, active internal bleeding, perispinal hematoma, or uncorrected coagulopathy present.

Adapted from Chest 2008;133:381–453.

Duration of Thromboprophylaxis
• Those at moderate–high risk of VTE should receive prophylaxis for entire hospitalization
• Extended thromboprophylaxis (28–35 d) for total hip or total knee arthroplasties, hip fracture surgery, or abdominal/pelvic surgery for cancer

Antithrombotics and Antiplatelets with Regional Anesthesia or Lumbar Punctures
• Wait times before epidural or dural punctures or prior to epidural catheter removal

> Wait 7 d after clopidogrel use; 8–12 h after SQ heparin; 10–12 h after bid prophylactic dose of LMWH; 18 hr after daily prophylactic dose of LMWH; 24 hr after therapeutic dose of LMWH; 36 hr after fondaparinux
- May perform neuraxial block, LP or remove epidural catheter if INR <1.5 on warfarin
- Start SQ heparin/LMWH ≥2 hr and fondaparinux 12 hr after epidural catheter removed
- Wait times after neuraxial anesthesia before initiation of antithrombotics
> Wait 6–8 hr before daily prophylactic LMWH started; 24 hr before bid prophylactic or therapeutic LMWH; 4 hr before SQ heparin; and 12 hr before fondaparinux started

References: Clev Clin J Med *2005;72:157;* Reg Anesth and Pain Med *2003;28:172;* Anesth Analges *2007;105:1540;* Chest *2008;133:381–453.*

PERIOPERATIVE MANAGEMENT OF THE DIABETIC PATIENT

- Minor surgery in Type II DM patients controlled with oral agents
> Hold oral agents on day of surgery
> Cover glucose >180 mg/dL with correction dose insulin
- Minor surgery in Type II DM patients controlled with insulin
> Normal insulin glargine the night prior or half dose NPH insulin the AM of surgery
> Restart the normal insulin regimen once patient is eating well after surgery
- Major surgery in Type II DM patients
> Hold oral agents and give half dose of NPH insulin the morning of surgery
> Start continuous insulin infusion prior to surgery and continue perioperatively
- Surgery in Type I DM patients
> Start 5% dextrose fluids at 100–125 mL/hr the morning of surgery
> Control glucose with a continuous insulin infusion perioperatively

Postoperative Diabetic Management
- Target glucose levels 100–180 mg/dL using an insulin infusion after major surgery
> Fewer infectious complications and lower mortality if glucose <220 mg/dL
- Transition to subcutaneous insulin once the patient is tolerating oral intake well

References: Diabetes Care *2004;27:553;* NEJM *2006;355:1903;* and Diabetes Care *2008; 31:512.*

INPATIENT MANAGEMENT OF PATIENTS USING CHRONIC CORTICOSTEROIDS

- Patients using more than 5 mg/day prednisone on a chronic basis are presumed to have a suppressed HPA axis and are at risk for secondary adrenal insufficiency
- These patients need "stress dosing" of corticosteroids during acute illness or surgery
> For mild–moderate acute illness (ward patient), give 2–3 × normal dose × 2–3 d, then maintenance
> For critical illness, give hydrocortisone 50–100 mg IV q8h × 5–7 d or until critical illness has resolved then taper back to maintenance dosing over 2–3 days

Table 6-6 Perioperative Management of Patients Taking Chronic Steroids*

Operation	Recommended management
Minor	Hydrocortisone[†] 25 mg/d divided bid × 1 d; then resume regular dose
Moderate	Hydrocortisone[†] 25 mg IV q8h × 24 hr; then 25 mg IV q12h × 24 hr; then regular dose
Major	Hydrocortisone[†] 50 mg IV q8h × 24 hr; then wean to regular dose over 2–3 d

* Indicated for steroid use equivalent to prednisone ≥20 mg/d for at least 3 wk or >5 mg/d chronically.
† Give first dose within 1–2 hr of the operation start time.
Adapted from *J Amer Coll Surg* 2001;193:678.

References: J Am Coll Surg *2001;193:678* and Crit Care Clin *2006;22:245*.

MANAGEMENT OF PATIENTS WITH PSYCHIATRIC SYMPTOMS

Table 6-7 Medications and Substances That May Cause Psychiatric Symptoms

Depression	Anxiety	Psychosis	Mania
Alcohol	Alcohol	Acyclovir	Anabolic steroids
Amantadine	Anticholinergic meds	Antiarrhythmics	Amantadine
Amphotericin B	Antipsychotics	Anticholinergic meds	Amphetamines
Asparaginase	β₂-agonists	Anticonvulsants	Antidepressants
Barbiturates	Bupropion	Antihistamines	Benzodiazepines
Benzodiazepines	Caffeine	Antiparkinson meds	Bromocriptine
Calcium channel blockers	Corticosteroids	Antipsychotics	Cimetidine
Clonidine	Decongestants	Antispasmodics	Cocaine
Corticosteroids	Digoxin	Busulfan	Corticosteroids
Estrogens	H₂-blockers	Carmustine	Decongestants
Hydralazine	Interferons	Ciprofloxacin	Dextromethorphan
Interferons	Neuroleptics	Colchicine	Isoniazid
Isotretinoin	Sympathomimetics	Corticosteroids	Levodopa
Methyldopa	SSRIs	Cyclosporine	Methylphenidate
Metronidazole	Theophylline	Cytarabine	Sympathomimetics
Opiates	Tricyclic antidepressants	Digoxin	
Procarbazine		Disulfiram	
Propranolol		Etoposide	
Thiazides		5-fluorouracil	
Vinblastine		Ifosfamide	
Vincristine		Interferons	
		Metoclopramide	
		Opioids	
		Pentamidine	
		Sympathomimetics	
		Tacrolimus	
		Vidarabine	
		Zalcitabine	
		Zidovudine	

Management of Delirium or Agitation in the ICU or in Postop Patients

- Refer to pp. 56–59 and 64–65 for management of abstinence syndromes and the poisoned patient
- Evaluate for hypoxia, hypercapnia, myocardial ischemia, CHF, electrolyte abnormalities, dehydration, seizures, intracranial bleed, drug withdrawal, infection, sleep deprivation, or uncontrolled pain; and treat any correctable abnormality
  - ➤ Pain: agents chosen based on degree of pain (pp. 7–11 and Tables 2-1, 2-2, and 2-3)
- Check medication list and discontinue all nonessential drugs
- Antipsychotics for severe delirium or combativeness
  - ➤ If QTc <450–500 msec, haloperidol load of 2–10 mg IV q 20–30 min until patient calm
    - ○ Continue 25% haloperidol loading dose q6h × 24 hr then taper over 48–72 hr
  - ➤ If QTc >450–500 msec, olanzapine 2.5–10 mg IM; then 2.5–5 mg IM in 1–2 hr if needed
- Lorazepam 0.5–2 mg IV q4h as needed for agitation refractory to antipsychotics
- Nonpharmacologic interventions: frequent reorientation; avoid restraints or catheters if possible; maintain hydration; minimize noise, light, and excessive stimulation; provide cognitively stimulating activities; early mobilization; use a scheduled pain protocol; and allow patient to wear glasses or hearing aids if sensory impairment is present

Management of Depressive Symptoms

- All antidepressant classes have similar efficacy and choice depends on the medical comorbidities, drug–drug interactions, and side effect profiles of different agents
  - ➤ Refer to Table 14-2 for antidepressant options
  - ➤ SSRIs, SNRIs, DNRIs, and TCAs all take 3–4 wk for maximal clinical efficacy
  - ➤ For elderly patients, "start low and go slow" is the rule for medication dosing
- Methylphenidate 5 mg PO bid–tid effective for treatment of apathetic depression in elderly inpatients; can be used as adjunct to SSRIs and for ventilator-dependent patients

Initial Management of the Catatonic Patient

- Catatonic patients usually have an underlying diagnosis of schizophrenia or depression
- Most common signs: mutism, immobility, stupor, posturing, negativism, staring, rigidity, catalepsy, automatic obedience, stereotypy, and echophenomena
- Rule out: thyroid, adrenal, autoimmune, and metabolic disorders, HIV, drug intoxication, structural CNS diseases, meningoencephalitis, and parkinsonism
- Treatment: lorazepam 2 mg IM q4h × 24 hours

Initial Management Options for Acute Mania

- Lithium 300–600 mg PO bid
- Valproic acid 250 mg PO tid
- Carbamazepine 200 mg PO bid
- Olanzapine 2.5–5 mg PO/IM bid

Table 6-8 Adverse Reactions of Neuroleptic Medications

Adverse reaction	Description	Management
Dystonic reaction	Sudden rigidity of jaw, neck, or eyes	• Diphenhydramine 50 mg IM bid • Benztropine 1–2 mg IM bid
Parkinsonism	Cogwheel rigidity, masked facies, pill-rolling tremor, paucity of movement	
Akathisia	"Ants in the pants," restlessness, and inability to sit still	• Lorazepam 1–2 mg PO bid • Propranolol 20 mg PO tid
Neuroleptic malignant syndrome: see p. 61 for description and management		
Torsades de pointes	QTc prolongation and polymorphic VT	• Magnesium 4 g IV • Treat hypokalemia

References: Clin Chest Med *2003;24:713;* J Clin Psych *2003;64:1410;* J Clin Psych *2000;61:750;* Am J Geriat Psych *2008;16:558;* Mayo Clin Proc *2003;78:1423;* Crit Care *2007;11:214;* Clin Neuropharm *2006;29:144;* and Am J Psych *2003;160:1233.*

MEDICAL COMPLICATIONS IN PREGNANCY

Cardiac Disease or Complications in Pregnancy
• Cardiac arrest
  ➢ CPR performed with a wedge under the right hip
  ➢ Remove all fetal monitoring leads prior to defibrillation
  ➢ Consider perimortem C-section within 4 min if initial resuscitation fails and there is a viable fetus
• Contraindications to becoming pregnant: severe pulmonary hypertension, severe left ventricular systolic dysfunction (LVEF <0.2), severe mitral or aortic stenosis, and Marfan syndrome with dilated aortic root or type A aortic dissection

Table 6-9 Mortality Risk in Patients with Cardiac Disease During Pregnancy

Cardiac disease groups	Mortality
Low risk: small left-to-right shunt through atrial or ventricular septal defect, or patent ductus arteriosus; mild pulmonic or triscuspid valve abnormalities; corrected tetralogy of Fallot; bioprosthetic valve; mitral valve prolapse without regurgitation; bicuspid aortic valve without stenosis; mild valvular regurgitation with normal LVEF	<1%
Intermediate risk: moderate mitral stenosis; large left-to-right shunts; mechanical prosthetic valve; severe pulmonic stenosis; moderate aortic stenosis; uncorrected coarctation of aorta; uncorrected cyanotic congenital heart disease; prior MI; LVEF <0.4; history of peripartum cardiomyopathy with normal LVEF	5–15%
High risk: Marfan syndrome with aortic root or valvular involvement; severe pulmonary hypertension; NYHA 3–4 CHF; severe aortic stenosis; history of peripartum cardiomyopathy with depressed LVEF	25–50%

LVEF = left ventricular ejection fraction; NYHA = New York Heart Association.
Adapted from *Clin Cardiol* 2003;26:135.

- Peripartum cardiomyopathy: defined by CHF with LVEF <0.45 occurring ≥36 gestational wk or within 5 mo postpartum in absence of other causes of heart failure
  - CHF treatment: furosemide diuresis; afterload reduction with hydralazine and nitrates antepartum or ACEI postpartum; β-blockers when CHF compensated
  - Consider cardiac transplantation if minimal improvement by 12 mo postpartum
- Tocolytic-induced CHF: occurs with magnesium, β-agonists, or nifedipine
  - Higher incidence with concurrent corticosteroid administration
  - Treatment: discontinue tocolysis, furosemide, oxygen +/− noninvasive ventilation
- Afib
  - Rate control: metoprolol, verapamil, or digoxin; DC cardioversion if unstable
  - Heparin/LMWH for duration of pregnancy if persistent or paroxysmal Afib
- MI in pregnancy
  - Medications safe in pregnancy: aspirin and clopidogrel; metoprolol titrated to resting HR 55–65 if BP allows; nitrates and morphine; heparin or LMWH
    - Thrombolytics are relatively contraindicated in pregnancy
  - PCI with bare metal stent placement is safe in pregnancy
  - Delay delivery for ≥2 wk after MI if possible; vaginal delivery preferred over C-section
- Hypertrophic cardiomyopathy
  - β-blockers for dyspnea or angina; and avoid fluid overload intrapartum
- Mitral stenosis
  - Bed rest, loop diuretics, and rate control with β-blockers or digoxin
  - Heparin or LMWH for Afib/Aflut
  - Balloon mitral valvuloplasty for hemodynamic compromise
  - Consider vacuum-assisted or forceps-assisted vaginal delivery
- Aortic stenosis
  - Presentation: dyspnea, angina, or syncope starting late second to early third trimester
  - Consider a percutaneous aortic balloon valvuloplasty for hemodynamic instability
  - Use extreme caution with spinal/epidural anesthesia due to marked vasodilatation
- Mechanical heart valves
  - Warfarin better than heparin/LMWH for preventing cardioembolic events
    - Warfarin causes an embryopathy if given during the first trimester
  - Heparin/LMWH <13 wk; warfarin 13–36 wk; then heparin/LMWH >36 wk

Hypertensive Emergencies in Pregnancy

- Severe preeclampsia: BP >160/110, >20 gestational wk, and ≥300 mg/d proteinuria
  - Treatment: start magnesium sulfate 4 g IV load then 2 g/hr infusion and deliver baby
- Hypertensive emergency <20 gestational wk: BP >160/110 with end-organ dysfunction
  - Treatment: hydralazine 5–10 mg IV q 15–20 min; labetalol 20–40 mg IV q 15–20 min (max 300 mg/d) or a drip at 0.5–2 mg/min; or IV nicardipine 5–10 mg/hr
  - IV nitroprusside 0.2–4 mcg/kg/min only in refractory hypertensive emergencies

- Hypertensive encephalopathy treatment: labetalol and nicardipine are preferred
- Myocardial ischemia: IV nitroglycerin 5–100 mcg/min

Pulmonary Complications During Pregnancy

- Amniotic fluid embolism
  - ➤ Typically occurs during labor, immediately postpartum, or after abdominal trauma
  - ➤ Presentation: sudden cardiovascular collapse, acute pulmonary edema, and often disseminated intravascular coagulation, altered mental status, and seizures
  - ➤ Treatment: mechanical ventilation with 100% oxygen, fluids, and inotropic support; FFP and cryoprecipitate for DIC; blood transfusions for active bleeding
    - ○ Consider a heparin drip for severe DIC **with thrombotic complications**
- Pulmonary embolism
  - ➤ D-dimer should be checked, but it may be elevated from pregnancy alone
  - ➤ A CT pulmonary angiogram and a V/Q scan have similar fetal radiation exposures
  - ➤ Duplex compression ultrasound of lower extremities to rule out DVT
  - ➤ Treatment: initiate IV heparin ×5 d; then transition to SQ heparin/LMWH
    - ○ SQ heparin q8h or LMWH q12h during pregnancy and until 6 wk postpartum
    - ○ Follow for thrombocytopenia; adjust LMWH based on anti-factor Xa levels
    - ○ Consider recombinant TPA for a massive PE with obstructive shock
- Acute respiratory distress syndrome (ARDS)
  - ➤ Lung-protective ventilation as outlined on p. 50
    - ○ May allow $PaCO_2$ to rise to 60 mmHg without detriment to the fetus
  - ➤ Avoid hyperventilation, as this will reduce uterine blood flow
  - ➤ Deliver baby as soon as possible once maternal condition stabilizes
- Severe pulmonary hypertension
  - ➤ Recommend hospitalization at 20 wk at a specialized referral center
- Cystic fibrosis
  - ➤ Poor maternal outcomes if pregravid FEV_1 <70% and FVC <60%
  - ➤ Consider termination of pregnancy if FEV_1 <50% or pulmonary HTN present
  - ➤ Treatments: inhaled and systemic antibiotics; chest physiotherapy; mucolytics; bronchodilators; nutritional support; and possibly supplemental oxygen
- Asthma exacerbation
  - ➤ Treatment is identical to that given in the nonpregnant state
  - ➤ Consider intubation for $PaCO_2$ >40–45 mmHg with increased work of breathing, maternal fatigue, fetal distress, or altered level of consciousness
  - ➤ Medications: bronchodilators, corticosteroids, oxygen +/– antibiotics

Table 6-10 Fetal Radiation Exposure and Effects with Different Radiological Tests

Test	Fetal radiation (mCy)	Radiation effect	Fetal radiation (mCy)
Chest x-ray	0.01	Teratogenicity	50–100
V/Q scan	0.2–1.4	Increased risk of childhood leukemia	20–50
CT pulmonary angiogram	0.1–0.9		
CT abdomen/pelvis	30–50		

Adapted from *Crit Care Med* 2005;33:1616.

Infectious Complications During Pregnancy

- Septic shock: follow guidelines on pp. 45–47 for severe sepsis and septic shock
  - APACHE II and SAPS II scores cannot be applied to critically ill pregnant pts
  - Antepartum sources include pneumonia, chorioamnionitis, and urosepsis
  - Postpartum: endomyometritis, septic abortion, or septic pelvic thrombophlebitis
  - Antibiotics: penicillins, cephalosporins, aminoglycosides, clindamycin, or carbapenems
  - Community-acquired pneumonia treated with ceftriaxone and a new macrolide
  - Dopamine or ephedrine (preferred vasopressors in pregnancy) → MAP ≥ 65 mmHg
  - Drotrecogin use has not been studied in pregnant patients; its safety is unknown

Hepatic Emergencies During Pregnancy

- HELLP syndrome: diagnostic criteria include hemolysis (LDH >600 IU/L, total bilirubin >1.2 ng/dL); AST and ALT 200–700 IU/L; and platelets <100,000/mL
  - Presentation: RUQ abdominal pain, nausea, vomiting, and preeclampsia
- Ruptured liver hematoma: occurs with severe preeclampsia, HELLP syndrome, or trauma
  - Contained hematomas should be managed conservatively
  - Unstable patients require an emergent laparotomy
- Acute fatty liver of pregnancy (AFLP): occurs during third trimester of pregnancy
  - Presentation: RUQ abdominal pain, nausea, vomiting, and fatigue
  - Labs: AST/ALT elevations up to 1000 units/L; elevated PT, PTT; decreased fibrinogen; renal failure; severe hypoglycemia; and bilirubin 1–10 ng/dL
  - Hyperbilirubinemia is more marked in AFLP, differentiating it from HELLP
- Treatment of both HELLP and AFLP is expeditious delivery of baby and supportive care

Neurologic Complications During Pregnancy

- Seizures
  - Eclamptic seizures: give magnesium 4 mg IV load then 2 g/hr; deliver baby
  - Status epilepticus: place patient supine with left lateral tilt
    - Lorazepam 2 mg IV q 1–2 min to max 0.3 mg/kg; phenytoin 18 mg/kg (up to 1 g) IV load at 50 mg/min → 100 mg IV q8h; then levetiracetam 1 g load → 500 mg IV bid
    - Intubation for ongoing seizures with propofol drip at 2–15 mg/kg/hr (if BP allows)
    - Pentobarbital 10–15 mg/kg IV load then 0.5–3 mg/kg/hr for refractory cases
- Intracranial hemorrhage treated same as in nonpregnant patients (see p. 54)
- Cerebral venous sinus thrombosis
  - Risk factors: advanced maternal age, hyperemesis, HTN, infection, and C-section
  - Presentation: headache, partial seizures, focal weakness, papilledema, and lethargy
  - Diagnosis: contrast-enhanced CT scan with bilateral infarcts and a "delta sign"
  - Treatment: heparin 80 units/kg IV load then 18 units/kg/hr × 5 d → SQ heparin or LMWH

Acute Renal Failure in Pregnancy

- Management: correct underlying etiology; avoid nephrotoxic meds; extreme caution with magnesium infusions; loop diuretic treatment only for volume overload
- Acute dialysis if: volume overload, uremia, or refractory hyperkalemia or acidosis

Trauma in Pregnancy
- Standard ATLS protocol, but maintain left lateral tilt in the patient
- Continuous fetal monitoring if >23–24 wk gestation for 4–6 hr, then intermittent
- Labs: FAST ultrasound scan for free fluid in abdomen, Kleihauer-Betke prep to screen for feto-maternal transfusion, and standard ATLS diagnostic studies
- Placental abruption or preterm labor occurs in 25–50% of major trauma
- Give Rhogam 300 mcg IM to all Rh-negative women

References: Crit Care Med 2005;33:S248-S397; Crit Care Med 2005;33:1616; Crit Care Med 2006;34:S208; Am J Med Sci 2008;335:65; J Fam Prac 2005;54:998; Heart 2004;90:450; and Curr Opin Crit Care 2005;11:430.

PERIOPERATIVE MANAGEMENT OF THE CIRRHOTIC PATIENT

Risk Factors for Surgery in Cirrhotic Patients
- Obstructive jaundice: hct >30%; total bili >11 mg/dL; malignancy; creatinine >1.4 mg/dL; albumin <3 g/dL; age >65 yr; AST >90 IU/L; and BUN >19 mg/dL
- Acute alcoholic hepatitis: elective surgery contraindicated
  ➢ Fulminant hepatic failure: consider candidacy for liver transplantation

Cirrhosis Scoring Systems Predictive of Postoperative Complications or Death
- Child-Turcotte-Pugh class and mortality rate for abdominal or cardiac surgery
  ➢ Nonemergent abdominal surgery: class A = 10%; class B = 30%; class C = 82%
  ➢ Emergent abdominal surgery: class A = 22%; class B = 38%; class C = 100%
  ➢ Elective cardiac surgery: class A = 0%; class B = 50%; class C = 100%
- MELD (Model for End-Stage Liver Disease) score
  ➢ Calculator available at: www.unos.org/resources/MeldPeldCalculator. asp?index=98
  ➢ Minimum lab value is 1.0 and max creatinine is 4 mg/dL; max score = 40
  ➢ For elective abdominal operations, 90-day mortality rate is: 10% if MELD score ≤8; 25% if MELD score 9–16; and 50% if MELD score >16
  ➢ 30-day mortality for nontransplant surgery increases 1% per point for MELD scores between 6 and 20 and 2% per point for scores above 20
  ➢ Recommend no nonemergent surgery if MELD score >15; consider surgery with close monitoring for MELD score 10–15; proceed with surgery for MELD score <10

Preoperative Management of Decompensated Cirrhosis
- Nutritional recommendations: intake of 1–1.5 g/kg/day of protein and B vitamins
- Coagulopathy: vit K 10 mg PO daily ×3 d helps coagulopathy from malnutrition
  ➢ Prolonged PTT is more predictive of bleeding risk compared with elevated INR
    ○ Recommend FFP transfusions to normalize PTT before an invasive procedure
- Thrombocytopenia: platelet transfusion if <50,000/mm³ before invasive procedures
- Ascites: aggressive preop management minimizes the risk of postop pulmonary complications or wound dehiscence
- Hyponatremia: fluid restrict to 1–1.2 L/d for serum sodium <125 mmol/L
- Hepatic encephalopathy: correct all metabolic abnormalities, avoid sedative/narcotics, and use lactulose 20–30 g PO q6–8h titrated to 3 loose BMs daily
- Substance abuse: patients should be sober for several months prior to elective surgery

Postop Care
- Consider enteral and parenteral nutrition initially after major surgery
- Platelet transfusion if surgical bleeding and counts <70,000/mm³
- Hepatic encephalopathy: lactulose titrated to 3 loose BMs/d; can add neomycin 1–3 gm PO q6h or rifaximin 400 mg PO tid for refractory cases

- Early mobility and ambulation
- DVT prophylaxis with intermittent pneumatic compression stockings

Contraindications to Liver Transplantation

- Active substance abuse; noncompliance with medical therapy; severe cardiovascular disease; uncontrolled systemic infection; extrahepatic malignancy; severe psychiatric or neurologic disorders; and absence of a splanchnic venous inflow system

References: Crit Care Med *2004;32:S106;* Am J Surg *2004;188:580;* Crit Care Med *2006; 34:S225; and* Gastroenterol Hepatol *2007;4:266.*

Section 7
Dermatology

DERMATOLOGIC EMERGENCIES IN THE HOSPITAL

Urticaria
- **Classification:** ordinary urticaria; physical urticaria; contact urticaria; and urticarial vasculitis
- **Duration of lesions:** ordinary urticaria (2–24 hr); physical urticaria (≤1 hr); contact urticaria (≤2 hr); and urticarial vasculitis (1–3 d), often leaving petechiae or bruise-like discoloration
- **Workup:** no investigation is needed for acute urticaria
  - Chronic urticaria (>6 wk): CBCD, full chemistry and thyroid panel, and ESR
  - Urticarial vasculitis: skin biopsy, C3 and C4 levels, and a small-vessel vasculitis screen
- **Treatment**
  - Discontinue any potential offending medications
  - Mild–moderate urticaria: first-generation or low-sedating antihistamines (H_1-blockers)
  - Severe urticaria: H_1- and H_2-blockers +/– doxepin +/–prednisone 30–60 mg/d × 3 d
  - Severe autoimmune chronic urticaria: consider plasmapheresis or IVIG
  - Urticarial vasculitis: prednisone 1 mg/kg/d × 7–14 d and taper over 2 wk

Angioedema
- **Clinical presentation:** cutaneous angioedema causes a nonpruritic, nonpainful, and nonerythematous localized swelling of the face, genitals, extremities, and trunk
  - Swelling of oropharynx and GI tract can cause life-threatening asphyxia or severe abdominal pain
- **Etiologies:** meds (ACEIs, ARBs, aspirin, azithromycin, barbiturates, β-lactams, carbamazepine, carisoprodol, chloral hydrate, clonidine, delavirdine, estrogens, fibrinolytic agents, fluconazole, fluoroquinolones, itraconazole, mebendazole, montelukast, NSAIDs, oxcarbamazepine, procainamide, rituximab, sulfa drugs, and rarely risperidone or paroxetine); C1 esterase inhibitor deficiency (if recurrent and without urticaria)
- **Therapy**
  - Discontinue any potential offending medications
  - Severe laryngeal edema: 1 : 1000 epinephrine 0.3 mL SQ/IM, H_1-blockers, and methylprednisolone 1–2 mg/kg/d divided q6h
  - Associated bronchospasm: nebulized $β_2$-agonist
  - C1 esterase inhibitor deficiency: acute therapy with C1 inhibitor concentrate or 3 units FFP
    - Epinephrine of **no benefit** for angioedema caused by C1 esterase inhibitor deficiency

Bullous Pemphigoid (BP)
- **Clinical presentation:** onset age >60 yr; pruritic, tense bullae on normal or erythematous base located on lower abdomen, inner thighs, groin, axillae, neck, and flexural aspects of arms/legs
- **Medication–induced BP:** furosemide, ACEIs, NSAIDs, penicillins, cephalosporins, spironolactone, fluoxetine, bumetanide, and penicillamine

- **Diagnosis:** histopathology and immunofluorescence of skin biopsy
- **Treatment:** mild cases require no treatment; the disease is self-limited and resolves in 2–5 yr
  - ➤ Moderate disease: clobetasol propionate or betamethasone dipropionate bid
  - ➤ Severe disease: oral prednisone 0.5–0.75 mg/kg/d
    - ○ Adjunctive meds: tetracycline 250–500 mg PO qid and nicotinamide 500 mg PO qid

Pemphigus Vulgaris (PV)

- **Clinical presentation:** onset age 30s to 50s; flaccid, fragile blisters and slowly healing, painful erosions on the skin and mucosa (conjunctiva, mouth, nose, vagina, penis, and labia)
- **Diagnosis:** histopathology and immunofluorescence of skin biopsy
- **Treatment**
  - ➤ Steroids: prednisone 15 mg PO daily (mild PV); 1 mg/kg PO daily (moderate PV); and 2 mg/kg PO daily (severe PV) until clinical improvement begins, then taper steroids
  - ➤ Adjunctive meds: oral azathioprine 50–100 mg/d or cyclophosphamide 50–100 mg/d
  - ➤ Recommend transfer to a burn care unit for extensive disease with denudation

Stevens-Johnson Syndrome (SJS)

- **Etiologies:** meds (acetaminophen, aspirin/salicylates, antibacterial sulfonamides, allopurinol, barbiturates, carbamazepine, chloroquine, cimetidine, cyclophosphamide, dactinomycin, dapsone, fluoroquinolones, gold, isoniazid, lamotrigine, methotrexate, nitrofurantoin, NSAIDs, penicillins, phenytoin, plicamycin, rifampin, and theophylline) or mycoplasma, HSV, or varicella infection
- **Clinical presentation:** fever, pain, and malaise followed by a vesiculobullous eruption with positive Nikolsky sign involving 2 mucosal sites or 1 mucosal site and a visceral manifestation
  - ➤ Mucosal sites: mouth, conjunctiva, and less likely the esophagus or respiratory tract
- **Diagnosis:** skin biopsy with histopathology
- **Treatment**
  - ➤ Discontinue any potential offending medications
  - ➤ Aggressive wound care, fluid, and electrolyte replacement
  - ➤ Early debridement of skin lesions and skin grafting for severe cases
  - ➤ Eye care: lubricating eye drops q1–2h; steroid or antibiotic eye drops may also help
  - ➤ Avoid urinary catheters
  - ➤ Give tetanus prophylaxis and use antibiotics only for documented infection
  - ➤ Adjunctive therapy: IVIG 0.4–1 g/kg/d × 4 d; or cyclosporine 5 mg/kg PO daily
  - ➤ Recommend transfer to a burn care unit if >10% body surface area (BSA) involved
  - ➤ Methylprednisolone 1–2 mg/kg/d IV × 5–7 d for moderate–severe cases is of uncertain benefit

Toxic Epidermal Necrolysis (TEN)

- **Clinical presentation:** most severe variant of SJS with at least 30% BSA involved
- **Etiologies and diagnosis:** same as for SJS

Table 7-1 Score for the Evaluation of Toxic Epidermal Necrolysis (SCORTEN) to Assess and Predict Mortality

SCORTEN variables	SCORTEN score	Mortality rate
Body surface area involved more than 10%	0–1	3.2%
Age more than 40 yr	2	12.1%
Presence of malignancy	3	32.4%
Heart rate >120 bpm	4	62.2%
Blood urea nitrogen (BUN) >28 mg/dL	5	85.5%
Serum glucose >252 mg/dL	6–7	95%
Serum bicarbonate <20 mmol/L	—	—

Adapted from *Arch Dermatol* 2003;139:26.

- **Treatment**
  - ➢ General treatment strategy for TEN same as SJS
  - ➢ Additional eye care: steroid eye drops and regular release of symblepharon
  - ➢ Adjunctive treatments of potential benefit: plasmapheresis, IVIG, or cyclosporine

Acute Burns

Table 7-2 American Burn Association Burn Center Referral Criteria for Adults

Chemical burns	Any burns with significant inhalation injury
Burns of face, hands, feet, genitalia, perineum, or major joints	Burn injury in pts with preexisting medical disorders that can complicate management
Any third-degree burns	Burns and concomitant trauma where the burn injury poses the greatest risk of death or morbidity
Electrical or lightning injuries	
Partial-thickness burns >10% BSA if >50 yr	Burn injury in pts requiring special social, emotional, or long-term rehabilitation services
Partial-thickness burns >20% BSA at any age	

Adapted from *Plast Reconstructive Surg* 2008;121:311e.

Treatment

- **Fluid resuscitation**
  - ➢ Burns involving >20% BSA should have aggressive fluid resuscitation
  - ➢ LR or isotonic saline 2–4 mL/kg/%BSA in first 24 hr; 50% of fluids in first 8 hr
  - ➢ Monitor bladder pressure every 4 hr to rule out abdominal compartment syndrome
  - ➢ Titrate fluid replacement to maintain a urine output ≥0.5 mL/kg/hr
- Placement of urinary catheters and nasogastric tubes in all patients with major burn injuries
- Early fiberoptic bronchoscopy to diagnose inhalation injuries for any patient at risk
- Nutritional support: early NG feeds started within 8–12 hr for all major burn injuries
- **Prophylaxis**
  - ➢ Stress ulcer prophylaxis: initiate a proton pump inhibitor or an H_2-receptor blocker

BURNS

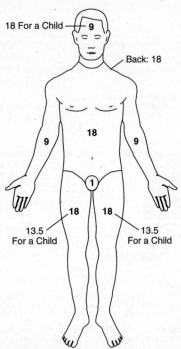

18 For a Child — 9

Back: 18

9   18   9

1

18   18

13.5
For a Child

13.5
For a Child

Figure 7-1 Rule of Nines Diagram for Burns

> DVT prophylaxis: initiate SQ heparin or low-molecular weight heparin
> Give tetanus prophylaxis if indicated
- **Wound care**
  > Leave blister overlying partial-thickness burns intact until definitive wound care done
  > Daily surgical debridement of second- and third-degree burns to level of healthy tissue
  > Escharotomies for all full-thickness circumferential burns of an extremity
  > Wounds covered with silver sulfadiazine
  > Definitive burn wound coverage typically with split-thickness skin grafts
- Aggressive pain control with opiate PCA
- Passive warming measures: use warmed IV fluids, a Baer Hugger, and heat lamps
- Early mobilization with physical therapy and occupational therapy
- **Indications for orotracheal intubation**
  > Patients with significant inhalation injuries
  > Large burns with anticipated need for large volume crystalloid resuscitation
  > Consider for major burn casualties who require air or ground transport

References: Crit Care Med *2008;36:S318;* Ann Allergy Asthma Immunol *2006;97:272;* J Burn Care *2008;29:269;* Drugs *2006;65:905;* Southern Med J *2008;101:186;* Drug Safety *2001;24:599;* Plast Reconst Surg *2008;121:311e;* J Burn Care Res *2008;29:257;* and Brit J Dermatol *2001;144:708.*

Section 8
Endocrinology

INPATIENT MANAGEMENT OF DIABETES

Table 8-1 Estimating Total Daily Insulin (TDI) Needs in Type 2 DM Based on BMI

Insulin resistance	BMI	Total daily insulin (units)
Normal	<25	Weight (kg) × 0.4 = # of units
High	25–30	Weight (kg) × 0.5 = # of units
Markedly high	>30	Weight (kg) × 0.6 = # of units

Adapted from *Diabetes Care* 2008;31:512.

Basal Insulin: Long-Acting Insulins (see Table 8-2)
- Start with 50% of TDI or 0.2–0.3 units/kg/d SQ given at the same time each day
- Increase dose 10–20% daily until fasting glucose <130 mg/dL

Prandial Insulin: Rapid-Acting Insulins (see Table 8-2)
- Option 1: start with 50% of TDI divided by 3 or 1 unit per 15 g carbohydrates consumed
- Option 2: insulin:carbohydrate ratio = 450/TDI to determine the grams of carbohydrate covered by 1 unit insulin (e.g., if TDI = 100 units, 1 unit insulin covers 4.5 g carbohydrate)
- Option 3: fixed dose regimen with 0.05–0.1 unit/kg/meal or 4–10 units/meal lispro
- Increase dose 10% until 2-hr post-prandial glucose <180 mg/dL

Correction Dose Insulin: Rapid-Acting Insulins (see Table 8-2)
- Used with basal insulin and prandial insulin to achieve better glycemic control
- Correction dose (CD) = (actual glucose − target glucose)/correction factor (CF)
  ➤ CF = 1700/total daily insulin (TDI)
  ➤ If glc = 200, goal = 100, and TDI = 34 units: CD = (200−100)/(1700/34) = 100/50 = 2 units

Table 8-2 Insulins

Insulin	Onset (min)	Peak (hr)	Duration (hr)
Rapid-acting insulins			
Lispro (Humalog)	15–30	0.5–2.5	3–6.5
Aspart (Novolog)	10–20	1–3	3–5
Glulisine (Apidra)	10–15	1–1.5	3–5
Short-acting insulins			
Regular (Humulin R)	30–60	1–5	6–10
Regular (Novolin R)	30–60	1–5	6–10
Intermediate-acting insulins			
Lente (Humulin L)	60–180	6–14	16–24
NPH (Humulin N)	60–120	6–14	16–24+
Long-acting insulins			
Glargine (Lantus)	70	—	24
Detemir (Levemir)	50–120	—	20–24

Other Medical Conditions Warranting Careful Glycemic Control
- Target glucose levels 100–180 mg/dL with insulin for the following conditions
  - ➤ Acute MI, severe sepsis or septic shock, and after an acute stroke
- Glycemic goals for medical or surgical inpatients on the general wards
  - ➤ Fasting and preprandial glucose 90–130 mg/dL and postprandial glucose <180 mg/dL

Transitioning from Parenteral to Subcutaneous Insulin
- Determine the total daily IV insulin requirement or estimate using Table 8-1
  - ➤ May be more accurately calculated using the last 8 hr of insulin and multiply by 3
- Use 80% of TDI to determine estimate for total daily subcutaneous insulin
  - ➤ Administer 50% as long-acting basal insulin (e.g., insulin glargine or detemir)
    - ○ Discontinue insulin drip 2 hr after SQ injection of insulin glargine or detemir
  - ➤ Administer 50% as prandial insulin (a rapid-acting insulin) divided by 3 with meals

Limitations of Oral Diabetic Agents for Inpatient Glycemic Control
- Sulfonylureas have a long half-life and cause hypoglycemia with erratic food intake
- Avoid metformin with IV contrast, CrCl <50 mL/min, or decompensated CHF
- Thiazolidinediones increase the risk of fluid retention and CHF
- No data for the use of GLP-1 receptor agonists (e.g., exenatide), amylin analogues (e.g., pramlintide), DPP-4 inhibitors (e.g., sitagliptin), or meglitinides in the hospital.

Nutritional Guidelines
- Diet is a modified carbohydrate diet with each meal containing 60 g of carbohydrates

References: NEJM 2006;355:1903; Diabetes Care 2004;27:553; Diabetes Care 2006;29:1955; Ann Intern Med 2006;145:125; JAMA 2008;300:933; and Diabetes Care 2008;31:512.

HYPERTHYROIDISM AND THYROID STORM

Etiologies of Hyperthyroidism
- Graves disease; toxic multinodular goiter; toxic nodule; hyperthyroid phase of thyroiditis; iatrogenic; TSH-secreting pituitary adenoma; struma ovarii; thyrotoxicosis factitia; metastatic follicular thyroid cancer; gestational trophoblastic disease; medication-induced: amiodarone, interferon-α, iodinated radiocontrast dyes; kelp and seaweed

Clinical Presentation of Hyperthyroidism
- **Signs:** diaphoresis, fine resting tremor, hyperreflexia, hyperdefecation, muscle weakness, diffuse goiter, irregular menses, infertility, insomnia, weight loss despite good appetite, poor concentration, moist smooth skin, onycholysis, hair loss, dependent edema, and tachycardia
- **Symptoms:** fatigue, weakness, nervousness, hyperactivity, irritability, insomnia, palpitations, heat intolerance, pruritus, exertional intolerance, dyspnea, and mood lability
- **Complications:** Afib, periodic paralysis, CHF, psychosis, and thyroid storm

Manifestations Characteristic of Graves Disease
- Ophthalmopathy: exophthalmos, lid retraction, lid lag +/–retrobulbar pain
- Infiltrative dermopathy: typically localized to the anterolateral aspect of the shin
- Radioactive iodine 123 (^{123}I) uptake scan with diffuse uptake; TSI-positive in 80% of patients

- Associated with autoimmune diseases: Type I DM, Addison disease, vitiligo, pernicious anemia, alopecia areata, myasthenia gravis, and celiac disease

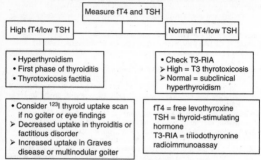

Figure 8-1 An Approach to Patients with Suspected Hyperthyroidism

Treatment Options for Hyperthyroidism

- If thyroid gland ≤2 × normal and soft, mild–moderate hyperthyroidism, children, or pregnant or lactating women, recommend using antithyroid drugs (ATDs)
  > Induction dose: methimazole 10–20 mg PO q8h or propylthiouracil 100–200 mg PO q8h
- Radioiodine ablation indications: thyroid >2 × normal or hard; multinodular goiter; Afib; high thyroid-stimulating immunoglobulin (TSI) titer; young man; or relapse after ATD therapy
- Subtotal thyroidectomy: pregnant patients with thyroid storm; severe exophthalmos intolerant of or refractory to ATDs; large goiter with compressive symptoms; a suspicious thyroid nodule; or relapse after ATDs and refusing ^{131}I therapy
- Propranolol is an adjunctive agent for tachycardia, tremors, and nervousness

Subclinical Hyperthyroidism

- Young, asymptomatic patient and non-nodular thyroid disease: follow
- Consider low-dose ATDs to normalize TSH if: symptomatic with osteoporosis or Afib; nodular thyroid disease; or >60 yr with TSH <0.1 mU/L
- If symptoms resolve with therapy, can consider ^{131}I radioiodine ablation

Management of Thyroid Storm

- Supportive care: fluid resuscitation with D5NS, thiamine and a multivitamin daily
- Find and treat precipitating cause (infection, MI, stroke, DVT, PE, or substance abuse)
- Antithyroid drugs: propylthiouracil 200–300 mg PO q6h or methimazole 20–30 mg PO q6h
  > Consider an initial load of propylthiouracil 600 mg PO (especially during pregnancy)
- Supersaturated potassium iodide (SSKI) 5 gtts PO q6h or Lugol's solution 4–8 gtts PO q6–8h; use at least 1 hr after ATDs

Table 8-3 Diagnostic Criteria for Thyroid Storm

Criteria	Points	Criteria	Points
Temperature (°F)		**GI–hepatic dysfunction**	
99–99.9	5	Absent	0
100–100.9	10	Diarrhea, vomiting, abd. pain	10
101–101.9	15	Marked unexplained jaundice	20
102–102.9	20	**Tachycardia**	
103–103.9	25	90–109	5
≥104	30	110–119	10
CNS effects		120–129	15
Absent	0	130–139	20
Mild agitation	10	≥140	25
Delirium, psychosis or ↑↑ lethargy	20	**Congestive heart failure**	
Seizures or coma	30	Absent	0
Atrial fibrillation		Mild	5
Absent	0	Moderate	10
Present	10	Severe	15
Precipitating event absent	0	**Precipitating event present**	10

A total score ≥45 is highly suggestive, 25–44 is possible, and < 25 is unlikely to be thyroid storm.
Adapted from *Endocrinol Metab Clin N Am* 1993;22:263.

- Propranolol 40–80 mg PO q6h or esmolol 50–100 mcg/kg/min IV
- Acetaminophen as needed for fever; avoid salicylates, as they can aggravate thyrotoxicosis
- Hydrocortisone 100 mg IV q8h or dexamethasone 2 mg IV q6h × 4 doses; especially if hypotensive

References: Endocrin Metab Clin N Am *2006;35:663;* J Clin Endo Metab *2007;92:3;* Obstet Gynecol Survey *2007;62:680;* and Lancet *2003;362:459.*

HYPOTHYROIDISM AND MYXEDEMA COMA

Etiologies of Hypothyroidism
- Thyroiditis syndromes (Table 8-4); post-thyroidectomy or postradioablation; panhypopituitarism; chronic iodine deficiency; medication-induced: amiodarone, antithyroid

Table 8-4 Thyroiditis Syndromes

Category	Hashimoto thyroiditis	Painless postpartum thyroiditis	Painful subacute thyroiditis	Painless sporadic thyroiditis	Painful suppurative thyroiditis
Onset	Usually 30–50 yr	≤4 mo postpartum	20–60 yr	Usually 30–40 yr	Children and 20–40 years
Anti-TPO antibodies	High titers in 90%	High titers	Low titer or absent	High titers	Absent
ESR	Normal	Normal	High	Normal	High
24-hr RAI ^{123}I uptake	Variable*	<5%	<5%	<5%	Normal or low

anti-TPO = anti-thyroid peroxidase antibody; ESR = erythrocyte sedimentation rate; RAI ^{123}I = radioactive iodine 123 uptake scan.
*Uptake is high in rare cases of hashitoxicosis, but usually is low.
Adapted from *NEJM* 2003;348:2646.

drugs, interferon-α, iodides, lithium, phenylbutazone, dopamine, glucocorticoids, octreotide, and sulfonylureas

Clinical Presentation of Hypothyroidism
- **Signs:** dry, yellow skin; coarse hair; hair thinning; delayed relaxation of reflexes; galactorrhea; growth failure; irregular menses; infertility; hypothermia; bradycardia; myxedema; mental impairment; poor concentration; eyebrow loss; deep, hoarse voice; constipation; weight gain; periorbital edema; and macroglossia
- **Symptoms:** cold intolerance, fatigue, weakness, myalgias, decreased libido, and confusion
- **Complications:** myxedema coma, pericardial effusion, heart block, hypertension infertility, dementia, ataxia, psychosis, and carpal tunnel syndrome
- **Labs:** hyponatremia, hyperlipidemia, and elevated creatinine phosphokinase

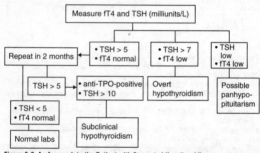

Figure 8-2 An Approach to the Patient with Suspected Hypothyroidism
TSH = thyroid-stimulating hormone; fT4 = free levothyroxine; anti-TPO-positive = anti-thyroid peroxidase antibody titer ≥1:1600.

Initial Management of Hypothyroidism
- Start full replacement dose of levothyroxine 1.6 mcg/kg/d for young, healthy adults
- Consider starting 1.3 mcg/kg/d levothyroxine in elderly patients or those with CAD

Management of Subclinical Hypothyroidism
- Levothyroxine for: TSH >10, α-TPO antibody-positive, infertility, or pregnancy
  - ➤ Titrate levothyroxine dose to achieve TSH levels 1–2.5 milliunits/L

Myxedema Coma
- **Clinical presentation:** CNS depression, hypothermia, hypoventilation, bradycardia, anorexia, nausea, abdominal pain, ileus, urinary retention, constipation, pericardial effusion, acute kidney injury, and potentially hypotension
- **Lab findings:** hyponatremia, anemia, elevated lactic acid and CK, and hyperlipidemia
- **Management**
  - ➤ Evaluate/treat precipitants (infection, CHF, stroke, trauma, MI, or hypothermia)
  - ➤ Intubation for inability to protect airway or ventilatory failure

> Passive rewarming with Baer Hugger, warm IV fluids, and heat lamps
> Volume resuscitation with D$_5$NS
> Levothyroxine 300–500 mcg IV load → 100 mcg IV daily → 1.6 mcg/kg PO daily
> Hydrocortisone 100 mg IV q8h × 2–3 d, then gradually taper over 5–7 d

References: Endocrinol Metab Clin N Am *2007;36:595;* Endocrinol Metab Clin N Am *2006;35:687;* J Intensive Care Med *2007;22:224;* and NEJM *2001;345:260.*

ADRENAL INSUFFICIENCY AND ADRENAL CRISIS

Table 8-5 Etiologies of Adrenal Insufficiency

Primary adrenal insufficiency	Secondary adrenal insufficiency
• Metastatic carcinoma of lung, breast, kidney, stomach, colon, or lymphoma	• Systemic glucocorticoid therapy >3 consecutive wk within the last yr
• Tuberculosis (Tb) or fungal infection	• Pituitary or hypothalamic tumors or postradiation or postsurgery
• Adrenoleukodystrophy	
• AIDS-associated infections*	• Lymphocytic hypophysitis
• Waterhouse–Friedrichsen syndrome	• Postpartum pituitary necrosis (Sheehan syndrome)
• Autoimmune adrenalitis	
• Adrenal hemorrhage/infarct	• Pituitary Tb, sarcoidosis, cryptococcosis, or histoplasmosis
• Antiphospholipid syndrome	
• Meds: etomidate, fludrocortisone, ketoconazole, megestrol acetate, phenobarbital, phenytoin, high-dose progestins, or rifampin	

*Most commonly HIV, cytomegalovirus infections, histoplasmosis, or mycobacterial infections.
Adapted from *Endo Met Clin N Am* 2006;35:767.

Symptoms of Adrenal Insufficiency (AI)
• Fatigue, malaise, weakness, poor memory, depression, psychosis, anorexia, postural dizziness, nausea/vomiting, abdominal pain, myalgias, arthralgias; also decreased libido (Secondary AI)
• Salt craving in primary adrenal insufficiency

Table 8-6 Signs and Typical Labs in Adrenal Insufficiency (AI)

Both types of AI	Primary AI	Secondary AI
• Unexplained fever	• Hyperpigmentation of palmar creases, extensor surfaces, and buccal mucosa	Pituitary lesions may exhibit:
• Hypotension or orthostatic hypotension		• Amenorrhea
• Hyponatremia	• Hyperkalemia	• Secondary hypothyroidism
• Hypoglycemia	• Nonanion gap acidosis	• Diabetes insipidus
• Mild hypercalcemia	• Possible vitiligo	• Sexual dysfunction
• Normocytic anemia		
• Eosinophilia		

Adapted from *NEJM* 2003;348:727.

Diagnosis of Adrenal Insufficiency in Acute Illness
• Overt AI likely if random cortisol <10–15 mcg/dL and unlikely if cortisol >34 mcg/dL
• A 250-mcg cosyntropin stimulation test can assess for AI if random cortisol 15–34 mcg/dL
> A cortisol rise <9 mcg/dL makes AI highly likely; an increase ≥16.8 mcg/dL excludes AI

Treatment of Presumed Adrenal Crisis
- 5% dextrose in isotonic saline infusion until normotensive
- Administer dexamethasone 4 mg IV and perform a cosyntropin stimulation test
- Hydrocortisone 100 mg IV q8h until results of cosyntropin stimulation test known

Maintenance Therapy of Adrenal Insufficiency
- Maintenance oral dose: prednisone 5–7.5 mg/d or hydrocortisone 20–25 mg/d
- Increase maintenance dose 2- to 3-fold during moderate illness or minor surgery
- Hydrocortisone 100 mg IV q8h during severe illness or for major surgery
- **Patients should wear a medic alert bracelet and medical identification card**

References: NEJM 2003;348:727; Ann Int Med 2003;139:194; Crit Care Med 2008;36:1937; Am J Resp Crit Care Med 2006;174:1319; Curr Opin Crit Care 2007;13:363; and Endo Met Clin N Am 2006;35:767.

CALCIUM DISORDERS

Hypercalcemia Etiologies (90% from hyperparathyroidism or cancer)
- Hyperparathyroidism (80–85% of cases from isolated parathyroid adenoma)
  - Most common cause of hypercalcemia; presentation is usually asymptomatic
  - Calcium level usually <11 mg/dL with an associated metabolic alkalosis
  - Elevated or inappropriately normal serum intact parathyroid hormone (iPTH) level
- Malignancy (bony metastases or humoral hypercalcemia of malignancy)
  - Breast, lung, lymphoma, thyroid, kidney, prostate, or multiple myeloma
  - Serum chloride/bicarbonate ratio low and calcium level often ≥13 mg/dL
  - 95% cases identified by history, exam, routine chemistries, complete blood count, CXR, and serum protein electrophoresis
  - Increased PTH-related peptide in humoral hypercalcemia of malignancy
- Other causes include: milk-alkali syndrome; vitamin A or D intoxication; granulomatous diseases (tuberculosis, coccidioidomycosis, berylliosis, or sarcoidosis) suggested by high serum calcitriol levels; thyrotoxicosis; familial hypocalciuric hypercalcemia (urine calcium/creatinine <0.01); Paget disease; adrenal insufficiency; pheochromocytoma; prolonged immobilization; and meds (thiazides, lithium tamoxifen, vitamin D, and gonadotropin-releasing hormone analogues, estrogens, androgens, caspofungin, theophylline, and teriparatide)
- ECG changes: shortened QT and prolonged PR intervals
- Complications: pancreatitis, nephrogenic diabetes insipidus, or nephrocalcinosis

Table 8-7 Clinical Presentation of Hypercalcemia

• Bone pain	• Diffuse abdominal pain, anorexia, nausea, and constipation
• Renal stones	• Lethargy, fatigue, depression, confusion, and cognitive impairment

Workup of Asymptomatic Primary Hyperparathyroidism
- Evaluate for osteopenia/osteoporosis: DEXA—bone mineral densitometry scan (DEXA = dual-energy x-ray absorptiometry)
- Rule out familial hypocalciuric hypercalcemia: check a fasting urine calcium/creatinine ratio as an outpatient once the patient is stable
- Check 25-hydroxy-vitamin D level: rule out secondary hyperparathyroidism
- Parathyroid Tc-99m sestamibi scan if surgery is being considered

Treatment Options for Asymptomatic Primary Hyperparathyroidism
- Daily PO intake of elemental calcium 1000–1200 mg and vitamin D 400–600 IU

- Parathyroid surgery indicated for any of the following: serum calcium is >11.2 mg/dL, nephrolithiasis, osteitis fibrosa cystic, CrCl <60 mL/min, bone density scan reveals a T-score ≤−2.5 at any site, age <50 yr, **or** medical surveillance is not desirable or possible
  - ➢ Surgery indicated for all patients with symptomatic primary hyperparathyroidism

Treatment of Hypercalcemic Crises (Serum calcium >13.5–14 mg/dL)
- Aggressive isotonic saline hydration 2–4 L/d with furosemide 20 mg IV q8–12h prn
- Hypercalcemia of malignancy: treat CA with surgery, chemotherapy, or radiation
  - ➢ Bisphosphonates: zoledronic acid 4 mg IV or pamidronate 90 mg IV over 4 hr
  - ➢ Refractory cases: gallium nitrate 100–200 mg/m² IV daily × 5 d
- Granulomatous disease: treat disease and hydrocortisone 100 mg IV q8h × 3–5 d → taper

Table 8-8 Hypocalcemia Etiologies

• Chronic renal failure	• Rhabdomyolysis	• Severe hypomagnesemia
• Hypoparathyroidism	• Respiratory alkalosis	• Massive transfusions
• Tumor lysis	• Acute pancreatitis	• Vitamin D deficiency
• Post-thyroidectomy	• Postparathyroidectomy from hungry bone syndrome	
• Meds: loop diuretics, phenytoin, phenobarbital, glucocorticoids, rifampin, aminoglycosides, and cisplatin		

Workup of Hypocalcemia
- Calcium (corrected) (g/dL) = calcium + [0.8 × (4 − serum albumin in g/dL)]
- If hypocalcemia etiology unclear, check intact PTH and 25-hydroxy-vitamin D levels

Clinical Presentation of Hypocalcemia
- Neuromuscular irritability (Chvostek sign and Trousseau sign), tetany, paresthesias, muscle cramps, and seizures
- Psychiatric disorders: psychosis, depression, and cognitive impairment
- ECG changes: prolonged QT interval +/−heart block

Treatment of Hypocalcemia
- 1.5–2 g of elemental calcium orally with meals daily divided bid–tid
- Add calcitriol 0.25 mcg PO daily–tid for hypoparathyroidism or vitamin D deficiency
- Calcium gluconate 1–2 g IV over 20 min for severe, symptomatic hypocalcemia

Reference: J Clin Endo Met 2009;94:335; NEJM 2004;1746–1751; Crit Care Med 2004;32:S146; Am J Med Sci 2007;334:381; and Am Fam Physician 2004;69:333–340.

HYPONATREMIA

Syndrome of Inappropriate Antidiuretic Hormone Secretion (SIADH)
- Diagnosis of exclusion; rule out hypothyroidism and adrenal insufficiency
  - ➢ Cerebral salt wasting is a hypovolemic state, and SIADH is a euvolemic condition
- Typically serum uric acid <4 mg/dL and blood urea nitrogen <10 mg/dL
- Causes: postoperative, severe pain, nausea or stress, CNS disorders (infection, bleeding, masses, multiple sclerosis, Guillain-Barré or Shy-Drager syndromes), lung process (pneumonia, pulmonary embolus, mechanical ventilation, asthma, cystic fibrosis, or lung cancer), delirium tremens, acute intermittent porphyria, psychosis, cancer, and medications (ACEIs [rare], barbiturates, bromocriptine, carbamazepine,

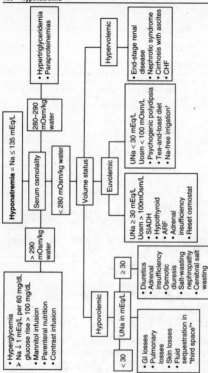

Figure 8-3 Workup of Hyponatremia

U = urine; Na = sodium; osm = osmolality; ARF = acute renal failure; SIADH = syndrome of inappropriate antidiuretic hormone secretion.

* As occurs in bowel obstruction, peritonitis, or acute pancreatitis.

† Used in hysteroscopy or transurethral resection of the prostate.

chlorpropamide, clofibrate, clozapine, cyclophosphamide, desmopressin, "ecstacy" abuse, general anesthesia, ifosfamide, indapamide, interferons, MAOIs, metformin, neuroleptics, nicotine, NSAIDs, opioids, oxcarbazepine, oxytocin, phenothiazines, SSRIs, tolbutamide, tricyclic antidepressants, valproic acid, vasopressin, or vincristine)

- Treatment: remove offending meds, treat underlying condition, and fluid restriction
  ➢ Infusions of isotonic saline alone usually worsens the hyponatremia of SIADH
  ➢ Consider demeclocycline 300–600 mg PO bid for treatment of chronic SIADH

Reset Osmostat (or "sick cell syndrome")

- Occurs with severe malnutrition, Tb, AIDS, alcoholics, terminal CA, and pregnancy
- Patients appropriately regulate serum osmolality around a reduced set point

General Guidelines for the Treatment of Hyponatremia

- Hypovolemic, hypotonic hyponatremia: use isotonic saline until euvolemic
- Hypervolemic or hypotonic, euvolemic hyponatremia: free water restrict to 750–800 mL daily in severe cases and 1000–1500 mL daily in mild–moderate cases
  ➢ Conivaptan 20 mg IV load then 20 mg IV infusion over 24 hr × 1–4 d
- Hypertonic saline +/–furosemide in the ICU for severe, symptomatic hyponatremia (lethargy, delirium, seizures, or coma) from any cause until Na ≥120 mEq/L
- IV fluid rate approximated by the following equation for the correction of hyponatremia or hypernatremia. Note: equation does not account for ongoing sodium losses or the effect of loop diuretics (e.g., furosemide use):

  ➢ Change in serum Na (after 1L infusate) $= \dfrac{[(\text{infusate Na} + \text{infusate K}) - \text{serum Na}]}{\text{Total body water (L)} + 1}$

  ➢ Total body water (L) = 0.6 × weight (kg) for men and 0.5 × weight (kg) for women
- Maximum correction of 1 mEq/L/hr; 8–10 mEq/L in 24 hr; and <18 mEq/L in 48 hr
  ➢ More rapid correction can lead to osmotic demyelination syndrome

References: NEJM 2007;356:2064; South Med J 2006;99:353; JAMA 2004;291:1963; Am Fam Physician 2004;69:2387; Am J Med 2007;120:S1; and Am J Med 2007;120:653.

HYPERNATREMIA

- **Etiologies**
  ➢ Hypovolemic hypernatremia
    ○ Extrarenal free water losses (skin, pulmonary, or gastrointestinal)
    ○ Renal causes: osmotic diuresis (mannitol/glucose); postobstructive diuresis
  ➢ Euvolemic hypernatremia
    ○ Diabetes insipidus: Uosm <300 mOsm/L with polyuria (>3 L urine output/d)
      ▪ Central DI: Uosm increases >50% after vasopressin 5 units SQ
      ▪ Nephrogenic DI if Uosm unchanged with vasopressin; causes include amyloidosis, myeloma kidney, lithium, foscarnet, or amphotericin B
    ○ Hypothalamic disorders (cancer, granulomatous diseases, or strokes)
  ➢ Hypervolemic hypernatremia
    ○ Mineralocorticoid excess: Conn syndrome or Cushing syndrome
    ○ Excessive sodium administration
- **Clinical features**
  ➢ Confusion, weakness, and lethargy; coma can occur in severe cases
- **Treatment**
  ➢ Central DI treated with vasopressin 0.1–1.2 mg/d PO divided bid–tid or DDAVP 10–20 mcg intranasally bid as needed

> - Initially volume replete dehydrated patients with isotonic saline
> - Once euvolemic, use the equation on p. 101 to correct sodium
>   - Max correction of 1 mEq/L/hr and replace free water deficit over 48–72 hr; if initial serum Na >170 mEq/L avoid correction to <150 mEq/L in first 48 hr
>   - Too rapid correction of hypernatremia can lead to cerebral edema.

References: NEJM 2000;342:1493 and South Med J 2006;99:353.

POTASSIUM DISORDERS

Hypokalemia Causes

- Decreased potassium intake (intake <40 mEq/d, extremely rare)
- Increased intestinal losses (vomiting, diarrhea, laxatives, sorbitol, or kayexalate)
- Increased renal losses (diuretics); hyperaldosteronism; hypomagnesemia; amphotericin B therapy; corticosteroid, fludrocortisone, or high-dose penicillins therapy; toluene intoxication ("glue sniffing"); osmotic diuresis (e.g., uncontrolled diabetes); Bartter syndrome; and Gitelman syndrome
- Type I (distal) or type II (proximal) renal tubular acidosis
- Increased cellular shift into cells: alkalosis; insulin; high-dose β-agonist; intoxication with caffeine, chloroquine, risperidone, or quetiapine; tocolytics; theophylline; and severe hypothermia
- Hypokalemic periodic paralysis (HPP)
- Increased blood cell production: post-therapy with vitamin B_{12}, folate, or granulocyte-macrophage colony-stimulating factor (GM-CSF)

Clues to Certain Etiologies of Hypokalemia

- Metabolic acidosis: renal tubular acidosis, chronic diarrhea, or toluene abuse
- Metabolic alkalosis and normotensive: vomiting (low urine chloride) or diuretics, Gitelman syndrome (↓ UCa) versus Bartter syndrome (↑/NL UCa) (UCa = urine calcium)
- Metabolic alkalosis and hypertension: Conn syndrome (hyporenin/hyperaldosteronism) or black licorice, ectopic corticotropin, or Liddle syndrome (hyporenin/hypoaldosteronism)
- Hypokalemic periodic paralysis: normal potassium between paralytic episodes, positive family history, thyrotoxicosis, normal acid–base status, transtubular potassium gradient <3.0, and urine potassium/creatinine ratio <2.5

Treatment of Hypokalemia

- IV KCl for ventricular arrhythmias, digoxin toxicity, paralysis, or severe myopathy
- PO KCl 20–80 mEq/d in divided doses for all other causes except:
  > - Hypokalemic periodic paralysis, which requires no more than 40 mEq PO KCl
  > - Renal tubular acidosis, which is treated with K-citrate or K-bicarbonate.

Hyperkalemia Causes

- Increased transcellular shift out of cells: metabolic acidosis, insulin deficiency, increased tissue catabolism, $β_2$-blockade, or digitalis intoxication
- Cellular breakdown: crush injury, severe burns, rhabdomyolysis, hemolysis
- Pseudohyperkalemia from hemolyzed blood specimen, marked leukocytosis, or marked thrombocytosis
- Decreased urinary potassium excretion: hypoaldosteronism, renal failure, ureterojejunostomy, and Addison disease
- Type IV renal tubular acidosis
- Meds: potassium, ACEIs, ARBs, NSAIDs, cyclosporine, heparin, amiloride, spironolactone, eplerenone, triamterene, pentamidine, and trimethoprim

- Tumor lysis syndrome

Treatment of Hyperkalemia (mnemonic CBIGKDrop)

C—calcium (1 ampule calcium gluconate IV for QRS widening from hyperkalemia)
B—bicarbonate (1 ampule sodium bicarbonate IV; most helpful if acidosis present)
I—insulin (10 units regular insulin subcutaneous or IV)
G—glucose (1 ampule of 50% dextrose unless patient already hyperglycemic)
K—kayexalate (15–30 g PO or 30–50 g in 100 mL enema PR)
D(rop)—dialysis

ECG Changes with Hypokalemia and Hyperkalemia

- Hypokalemia: ST depression → U waves
- Hyperkalemia: peaked T waves → PR prolongation → QRS widening, and p waves disappear → sinusoidal pattern

References: NEJM 1998;339:451–458; Crit Care Clinics 2002;18:273–288; and Arch Int Med 2004;164:1561–1566.

HYPOPITUITARISM

Table 8-9 Causes of Adult-Onset Hypopituitarism

Pituitary tumors	Pituitary apoplexy	Peripituitary lesions: meningioma, glioma, craniopharyngioma, brain mets
Pituitary surgery	Sheehan syndrome	
Pituitary radiotherapy	Head trauma	Pituitary infections: syphilis, Tb, or fungal
Subarachnoid hemorrhage	Infiltrative disorders: sarcoidosis, histiocytosis X, hemochromatosis, or lymphocytic hypophysitis	

Adapted from *Pituitary* 2005;8:183.

Table 8-10 Symptoms of Adult-Onset Hypopituitarism

Deficiency syndrome	Clinical presentation
Corticotrophs	Fatigue, weakness, dizziness, nausea, vomiting, anorexia, weight loss, hypoglycemia, and shock (in severe cases)
Thyrotropin	Fatigue, cold intolerance, constipation, weight ↑, hair loss, dry/coarse skin, bradycardia, hoarseness, slow cognition, hypothermia
Gonadotropin	women: amenorrhea, infertility, loss of libido, and osteoporosis men: ↓ libido, erectile dysfunction, hair loss, ↓ muscle/bone mass
Growth hormone	↓ muscle mass, central obesity, fatigue, weakness, premature atherosclerosis, and decreased quality of life

Adapted from *Pituitary* 2005;8:183.

Workup of Suspected Hypopituitarism

- Corticotroph deficiency: AM cortisol <3.5 mcg/dL or post-stimulation cortisol <18 mcg/dL after 250 mcg cosyntropin; and ACTH level low/low normal
- Thyrotrope deficiency: TSH levels low or low-normal and fT4 levels low
- Gonadotroph deficiency: LH and FSH levels low; women—estradiol low; men—testosterone low
- Somatotrope deficiency: GH and IGF-1 levels low or inappropriately normal
- Lactotroph function: prolactin levels high if stalk compression or prolactinoma
- Visual field testing as a sign of optic chiasm compression
- MRI of pituitary in all patients with confirmed hypopituitarism
- DEXA (bone mineral densitometry) at baseline and every 2 years

Replacement Dosing for Hypopituitarism

- Glucocorticoids: hydrocortisone 15 mg q AM and 10 mg q PM; or prednisone 5–7.5 mg/d
- Thyroid: levothyroxine 1.6 mcg/kg PO daily and titrate to normalize fT4 levels
- Hypogonadism in premenopausal women: 35 mcg ethinyl estradiol oral contraceptive pills
- Hypogonadism in men: injectable or transdermal testosterone replacement
- Growth hormone deficiency: treatment only after consultation with an endocrinologist
- Central DI: DDAVP 10–20 mcg intranasally bid; or vasopressin 0.1–1.2 mg/day PO divided bid–tid

References: Postgrad Med J *2006;82:259* and Pituitary *2005;8:183.*

Section 9
Gastroenterology

UPPER GASTROINTESTINAL BLEEDING (UGIB)

Causes of UGIB
- Peptic ulcer disease (30–50%); varices (10–30%); gastritis (10–15%); Mallory-Weiss tear (10–20%); esophagitis (5–10%); angiodysplasia (5%); and malignancy (2%)

Preendoscopy Clinical Predictors of Poor Outcome with UGIB
- Age >60 yr; cirrhosis; renal failure; cardiopulmonary disease; SBP <100 mmHg; concurrent sepsis; APACHE II score ≥11; presence of hematemesis, hematochezia, bright red nasogastric aspirate; or presence of coagulopathy, thrombocytopenia, or Hgb ≤8 g/dL

Glasgow-Blatchford Criteria for Low-Risk UGIB Suitable for Outpatient Management
- BUN <18 mg/dL; Hgb ≥13 g/dL (men) or ≥12 g/dL (women); SBP ≥ 110 mmHg; HR <100 bpm; and absence of melena, syncope, current or history of acute/chronic liver disease or heart failure
  ➤ Endoscopic intervention required in 0.5% of these patients and no risk of rebleeding or death

Table 9-1 Endoscopic Findings as Predictors of Outcome for Peptic Ulcers

Findings	Rebleeding risk	Surgery needed	Mortality risk
Clean base	5%	0.5%	2%
Flat spot	10%	6%	3%
Adherent clot	22%	10%	7%
Visible vessel	43%	34%	11%
Bleeding vessel	55%	35%	11%

Adapted from *NEJM* 1994;331:717.

Table 9-2 Rockall Scoring System for Upper Gastrointestinal Bleeds

Score	0	1	2	3
Age (yrs)	<60	60–79	≥80	—
Vitals	HR <100	HR ≥100	SBP <100	—
	SBP ≥100	SBP ≥100		
Comorbidities	None	—	Chronic heart or lung disease	Renal or liver failure; metastatic CA
Endoscopic findings	Mallory-Weiss No lesion/no SRH	All other diagnoses	Malignant lesion of upper GI tract	—
SRH	Clean base or dark spot on ulcer base	—	Adherent clot; visible or bleeding vessel	—

Rockall score	Rebleeding	Mortality	Rockall score	Rebleeding	Mortality
0–2	4.3%	0.1%	6	29%	15%
3–4	13%	3%	7	40%	20%
5	17%	8%	≥8	48%	40%

SRH = stigmata of recent hemorrhage (adherent clot, visible vessel, or bleeding vessel).
Adapted from *Lancet* 1996;347:1138.

Initial Treatment of Upper GI Bleeds

- Aggressive IV fluid resuscitation with isotonic saline or PRBC transfusions
- Platelet transfusion for platelet <50 K/µL
- Correct coagulopathy with FFP +/− vitamin K (until PTT normalizes in cirrhotic patients)
- Proton pump inhibitors IV bid (esomeprazole, lansoprazole, or pantoprazole) or as a continuous infusion (e.g., pantoprazole 80 mg IVP then 8 mg/hr infusion)
  - ➤ Continue PO bid × 4–8 weeks for peptic ulcer disease
  - ➤ Assess for *H. pylori* infection and treat if present

Gastroesophageal Variceal Bleeds

- Octreotide 50 mcg IV bolus, then infuse at 50 mcg/hr × 3–5 d for variceal bleeds
- Antibiotic prophylaxis × 7 d: decreases risk of spontaneous bacterial peritonitis or variceal rebleeding
- Endoscopic variceal ligation (EVL) or sclerotherapy if ligation not possible
  - ➤ Serial EVL every 3 wk until varices are obliterated
- β-blockers: propranolol or nadolol titrated to decrease resting heart rate 25%
- Nitrates: isosorbide mononitrate 30 mg PO daily; added to serial endoscopic variceal ligation and β-blockers
- Transjugular intrahepatic portosystemic shunt for gastric varices or recurrent esophageal variceal bleeds

Duration of Inpatient Observation

- None for Mallory-Weiss tears, gastritis, esophagitis, or clean ulcer base; 1 d for red spot on ulcer; 1–2 d for adherent clots; 3 d for visible or bleeding vessels treated endoscopically

References: J Clin Gastro 2007;41:559; Curr Opin Crit Care 2006;12:171; Arch Int Med 2007;167:1291; Lancet 2009;373:42; Gastro Clin N Am 2005;34:607; and NEJM 2001;345:669.

LOWER GASTROINTESTINAL BLEEDING (LGIB)

Causes of LGIB

- Diverticulosis; angiodysplasia; infectious or ischemic colitis; inflammatory bowel disease; hemorrhoids; UGIB; or malignancy

Risk Factors (RFs) for Poor Outcomes in LGIB

- SBP ≤115 mmHg; HR ≥100 bpm; syncope; nontender abdominal exam; hematochezia during first 4 hr of evaluation; history of aspirin or clopidogrel use; initial Hct ≤ 35%; and >2 active medical comorbidities
- Risk of severe bleeding: low (0 RFs; <10%); medium (1–3 RFs; 45%); high (>3 RFs; 80%)

Management of Lower Gastrointestinal Bleeding

- Bowel rest and aggressive fluid resuscitation with isotonic saline or PRBC transfusions
- FFP for coagulopathy if INR >1.5 or PTT elevated >1.5 × upper limit of normal
- Platelet transfusion if platelets <50 K/µL
- Treatment of uncontrollable LGIB: angiography with selective embolization versus surgery

References: Clev Clin J Med 2007;74:417; Surg Endosc 2007;21:514; Eur Radiol 2008;18:857; and Best Pract Res Clin Gastro 2008;22:295.

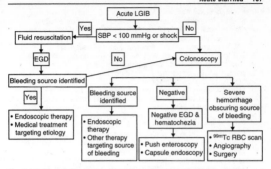

Figure 9-1 Suggested Evaluation of Acute Lower Gastrointestinal Bleeding (LGIB)
Source: Adapted from *Best Pract Res Clin Gastro* 2008;22:295.

ACUTE DIARRHEA

Clinical Presentation
- Acute diarrheal illness: ≥3 loose bowel movements/d (<2 weeks duration)
- Most cases are self-limited, viral (rotavirus or norovirus) etiology, and duration <48 hr

History
- **Clinical features suggesting viral gastroenteritis:** nausea, vomiting, watery diarrhea, mild–moderate abdominal pain, <6 stools/d, and duration <7 d
- **Clinical features worrisome for bacterial gastroenteritis:** fever >101.3°, voluminous or bloody diarrhea, >6 stools/d, severe abdominal pain, duration >7 d, tenesmus, hemolytic–uremic syndrome, immunocompromised state, or presence of fecal leukocytes or fecal lactoferrin
- Recent travel to developing areas (especially Latin America, Southern Asia, and Africa)
  ➢ 80% of traveler's diarrhea is bacterial (*E. coli* > *Campylobacter jejuni*)
- Recent contact with amphibians, reptiles, or ducklings (salmonella)
- Daycare or nursing home client or worker (viral, giardia, or shigella)
- Recent ingestion of undercooked eggs, beef, or poultry or old dairy products (campylobacter or salmonella) or shellfish ingestion (vibrio or norovirus)
- Recent antibiotics in last 2 months or chemotherapy (*Clostridium difficile* colitis)
- Medical conditions: immunocompromised, HIV-positive, or prior gastrectomy
- Med side effect: antacids, antibiotics, colchicine, laxatives, orlistat, and sorbitol

Workup Based on Category of Diarrhea
- No testing if diarrhea <3 d, no dehydration, fever <101.3°, **and** no blood/pus in stool

- **Community-acquired diarrhea (CAD) or traveler's diarrhea (TD)**
  - ➤ Stool for *Clostridium difficile* toxin if recent antibiotics or chemotherapy
  - ➤ Stool studies if clinical features consistent with bacterial etiology as above
    - ○ Stool culture for salmonella, shigella, campylobacter, or yersinia
    - ○ Stool for ova and parasites if giardia or amebiasis suspected
  - ➤ Test for *E. coli* 0157:H7 and shiga toxin if hemolytic–uremic syndrome present
  - ➤ Stool cultures for vibrio if recent ingestion of shellfish
- **Nosocomial diarrhea** (onset after 72 hr of hospitalization)
  - ➤ Stool for *Clostridium difficile* toxin
  - ➤ Check for salmonella, shigella, campylobacter, and/or *E. coli* 0157:H7 if immunocompromised, neutropenic, or suspected systemic enteric infection
- **Persistent diarrhea** (>7 d)
  - ➤ Check all stool studies **prior to** barium/contrast studies (or wait 14 d after)
  - ➤ Check fecal leukocytes as screen for inflammatory diarrhea
  - ➤ Consider stool studies for giardia, cryptosporidium, cyclospora, and isospora
  - ➤ If HIV-positive, add stool for microsporidia, blood cultures for *Mycobacterium avium complex*, and consider flexible sigmoidoscopy

Treatment of Acute Infectious Diarrhea
- IV hydration with isotonic saline or lactated Ringer solution if patient dehydrated
- Antimotility agents if patients are nontoxic and there is **absence** of fever, blood in stool, no fecal leukocytes, and no traveler's diarrhea; use loperamide or bismuth subsalicylate
- Probiotics (lactobacilli or saccharomyces) may decrease diarrhea severity and duration
- Empiric antibiotics for bacterial community-acquired or traveler's diarrhea
  - ➤ Rifaximin 200 mg PO tid × 3 d is preferred for afebrile, nondysenteric TD
  - ➤ Oral ciprofloxacin or levofloxacin × 5 d for CAD; × 1–3 d an option for TD
- Empiric treatment for severe nosocomial diarrhea (presumptive *C. difficile* colitis)
  - ➤ Mild–moderate disease: metronidazole 500 mg PO tid × 10 d
  - ➤ Severe disease: vancomycin 125 mg PO qid × 10 d
    - ○ Two of following: T >101°F; age >60 yr; albumin <2.5 mg/gL; or WBC >15°K cells/mm^3; or colonic distension on plain films or CT scan of abdomen
  - ➤ Contact isolation and careful handwashing using soap after contact with patient

References: NEJM 2004;350:38; Gastroenterol Clin N Am 2003;32:1249; Gastroenterol Clin N Am 2006;35:219–273, 337–353; J Emer Med 2002;23:125; Curr Opin Pharm 2005;5:559; NEJM 2008;359:1932; and Clin Infect Dis 2008;46:S32.

HEPATITIS

Classification
- **Hepatitis** is classified into cholestatic, hepatocellular injury, or infiltrative patterns.
  - ➤ **Cholestasis:** increased alkaline phosphatase > increased liver transaminases
  - ➤ **Hepatocellular injury:** increased liver transaminases > increased alkaline phosphatase
  - ➤ **Infiltrative diseases of the liver:** markedly increased alkaline phosphatase with low bilirubin

Table 9-3 Causes of Hepatitis

Cholestatic pattern	Infiltrative diseases affecting liver

Cholestatic pattern
- Gallstones
- Hepatocellular carcinoma
- Primary biliary cirrhosis
- Primary sclerosing cholangitis
- Venoocclusive disease
- Budd-Chiari syndrome

Med-induced cholestasis
- allopurinol
- amoxicillin-clavulanate
- anabolic steroids
- arsenicals
- azathioprine
- benzodiazepines
- carbamazepine
- chlorpromazine
- clindamycin
- clopidogrel
- cyclosporine
- cyproheptadine
- erythromycin
- estrogens
- felbamate
- fluoroquinolones
- fluoxetine
- flutamide
- glucocorticoids
- gold
- H$_2$-blockers
- haloperidol
- irbesartan
- mercaptopurine
- methimazole
- methotrexate
- mirtazapine
- naproxen
- niacin
- nitrofurantoin
- oral contraceptives
- penicillamine
- phenothiazines
- propoxyphene
- propylthiouracil
- pyrazinamide
- sulfasalazine
- sulfonylureas
- sulindac
- terbinafine
- tetracycline
- tricyclic antidepressants
- trimethoprim-sulfamethoxazole

Infiltrative diseases affecting liver
- Sarcoidosis
- Tuberculosis
- Deep fungal infections
- Hepatocellular carcinoma
- CA mets to the liver
- Leukemic infiltrate
- Lymphoma

Herbal hepatotoxins
- Amanita mushrooms
- Chaparral leaf
- Comfrey
- Germander
- Gordolobo herbal tea
- Greasewood
- Jin bu huán
- Kava kava
- Margosa oil
- Mate tea
- Mistletoe
- Oil of cloves
- Pennyroyal (squawmint)
- Skullcap
- Valerian root
- Yerba herbal tea

Conditions causing hepatocellular injury
- Alcoholic hepatitis
- Autoimmune hepatitits
- Chronic viral hepatitis
- Nonalcoholic steatohepatitis (diabetes and obesity)
- Congestive hepatopathy
- Wilson disease
- Hemochromatosis
- α_1-antitrypsin deficiency
- Ischemic hepatitis

Med-induced hepatocellular injury
- acarbose
- acetaminophen
- allopurinol
- amiodarone
- ACEIs
- aspirin/salicylates
- baclofen
- bupropion

- carmustine
- chlorpropamide
- cyclophosphamide
- dantrolene
- dapsone
- diclofenac
- fluconazole
- fluoxetine
- griseofulvin
- halothane
- heparin
- hydralazine
- isoniazid
- ketoconazole
- labetalol
- losartan
- MAOIs
- methotrexate
- methyldopa
- minocycline
- mithramycin
- NSAIDs
- nefazodone
- nevirapine
- nifedipine
- nitrofurantoin
- omeprazole
- paroxetine
- penicillins
- phenobarbital
- phenytoin
- piroxicam
- primidone
- procainamide
- pyrazinamide
- quinidine or quinine
- rifampin
- risperidone
- ritonavir
- sertraline
- statins
- stavudine
- sulfonamides
- tamoxifen
- thiazolidinediones
- trazodone
- valproic acid or divalproate
- venlafaxine
- verapamil
- zidovudine

Adapted from *NEJM* 2006;354:731–739; *Gastroenterology* 2002;123:1364–1384; and *Am Fam Physician* 2005;71:1105–1110.

Management of Severe Acute Alcoholic Hepatitis (AAH)

* Severe AAH: Glasgow alcoholic hepatitis score ≥9 or Maddrey's discriminant score >32
* Calculate MELD score at www.unos.org/resources/MeldPeldCalculator.asp?index = 98 (MELD calculator is used to assess mortality risk of patients with decompensated cirrhosis)
* Possible mortality benefit of PO prednisone 40 mg/d or prednisolone 32 mg/d × 28 d
  ➢ Glucocorticoids contraindicated for acute GI bleed, sepsis, renal failure, or pancreatitis
* Several studies suggest that pentoxifylline 400 mg PO tid is as effective as corticosteroids

Table 9-4 Glasgow Alcoholic Hepatitis Score

Parameters	1 point	2 points	3 points
Age	<50 yr	≥50 yr	—
WBC (10^9/L)	<15	≥15	—
BUN (mmol/L)	<5	≥5	—
INR	<1.5	1.5–2	>2
Bilirubin (mg/dL)	<1.4	1.4–2.8	>2.8

Adapted from *Gut* 2005;54:1057.

References: J Clin Gastro 2006;40:833 and *Aliment Pharmacol Ther 2007;27:1167.*

CIRRHOSIS

Etiologies of Cirrhosis in Adults in the United States

* Listed in order of prevalence: alcohol; hepatitis C or B virus; nonalcoholic steatohepatitis (from obesity or diabetes); hemochromatosis; primary biliary cirrhosis; Wilson disease; α_1-antitrypsin deficiency; and autoimmune hepatitis

Diagnosis of Cirrhosis

* Gold standard is a percutaneous liver biopsy; presumptive diagnosis by abnormal labs, exam, and imaging (ultrasound or radionuclide liver/spleen scan)

Table 9-5 Child-Turcotte-Pugh Scoring System for Cirrhosis Classification

Categories	1 point	2 points	3 points
Albumin (g/dL)	>3.5	2.8–3.5	<2.8
Bilirubin (mg/dL)	<2.0	2.0–3.0	>3.0
International Normalized Ratio	<1.7	1.7–2.3	>2.3
Presence of ascites	None	Diuretic-controlled	Diuretic-resistant
Encephalopathy	None	Grade 1–2 (mild)	Grade 3–4 (severe)

Class A = 5–6 points; Class B = 7–9 points; and Class C = ≥10 points.
1- and 2-yr mortality rates: Class A, 0% and 15%; Class B, 20% and 40%; Class C, 55% and 65%.
Adapted from *Crit Care Med* 2006;34:S225.

Clinical Features That May be Present in Cirrhosis

* General: muscle wasting, fetor hepaticus, anorexia, and testicular atrophy
* Skin: jaundice, spider angiomata, pruritus, and palmar erythema
* Thorax: gynecomastia and pleural effusion (hepatic hydrothorax)
* Extremities: Dupuytren contracture, white nails, and clubbing
* Abdomen: ascites, caput medusae, and splenomegaly
* Neurologic: confusion, decreased level of consciousness, and asterixis

Workup of Cirrhosis

- Labs: complete blood count, CHEM-7, liver panel, prothrombin time, and α-fetoprotein
- Labs to consider: hepatitis B and C virus serologies; iron studies; antimitochondrial, antinuclear, and antismooth muscle antibodies; serum ceruloplasmin; and α_1-antitrypsin level
- A percutaneous liver biopsy is indicated if the diagnosis is equivocal
- Imaging studies: abdominal ultrasound with Doppler of portal vein blood flow

Complications of Cirrhosis (any complication indicates decompensated cirrhosis)

- **General management of cirrhotic ascites**
  - ➢ Dietary restriction to 1–2 g sodium daily is essential for successful control
  - ➢ Consider fluid restriction if serum Na $\leq$125 mEq/L
  - ➢ Avoid aspirin, NSAIDs, and Cox-2 inhibitors; no role for bed rest
- **Management of moderate-volume cirrhotic ascites**
  - ➢ Spironolactone 50–200 mg PO q AM or amiloride 5–10 mg PO daily
- **Management of large-volume cirrhotic ascites**
  - ➢ Begin spironolactone 100 mg PO q AM and furosemide 40 mg PO q AM
  - ➢ Double dosages q 3–5 d until urine Na > urine K and weight loss 1 lb/d or maximal doses of spironolactone 400 mg PO q AM and furosemide 160 mg PO q AM
  - ➢ Monitor for encephalopathy, renal insufficiency, and electrolyte imbalances
- **Management of refractory ascites (diuretic-resistant ascites)**
  - ➢ Large-volume paracentesis q 2–4 wk +/– infusion of 8–10 g albumin for each liter of ascitic fluid if more than 5 liters of ascitic fluid is removed
  - ➢ Alternative is a transjugular intrahepatic portosystemic shunt (TIPS procedure)
    - ○ Contraindications to TIPS: portosystemic encephalopathy, CHF, pulmonary hypertension, multiple hepatic cysts, active infection, biliary obstruction, hepatic or portal vein thrombosis, central hepatoma, severe thrombocytopenia, or coagulopathy
  - ➢ Recommend referral of patients with ascites for liver transplantation (60–70% 5-yr mortality)
- **Spontaneous bacterial peritonitis (SBP)**
  - ➢ **Clinical features:** abdominal pain, fever, encephalopathy, or asymptomatic (10%)
  - ➢ **Diagnosis:** ascitic fluid neutrophils $\geq$250/mm^3 or monomicrobial bacterial growth
  - ➢ Secondary bacterial peritonitis if ascitic fluid white blood count >10,000/µL, glucose <50 mg/dL, LDH >250 U/L, protein >1 g/dL, alkaline phosphatase >240 units/L, carcino-embryonic antigen (CEA) >5 ng/mL, or polymicrobial Gram stain or culture growth
- **SBP treatment:** cefotaxime 2 g IV q8h or ceftriaxone 2 g IV daily $\times$ 5–7 d if uncomplicated or 10–14 d if complicated SBP or positive blood cultures
  - ➢ Albumin 1.5 g/kg IV on day 1 then 1 g/kg IV on day 3 had a 19% decrease in absolute mortality and decreases the risk of hepatorenal syndrome
- **SBP prophylaxis:** trimethoprim-sulfamethoxazole DS 1 tab PO daily, norfloxacin 400 mg PO daily, or ciprofloxacin 750 mg PO weekly
  - ➢ Indicated for prior SBP, if ascitic fluid protein <1 g/dL, or Tbili >2.5 mg/dL.
  - ➢ Norfloxacin 400 mg PO bid or ofloxacin 400 mg IV daily $\times$ 7 d for acute variceal bleed; improves survival and decreases risk of SBP or variceal rebleed

- **Gastroesophageal variceal bleed**
  - Octreotide 50 mcg × 1 → 50 mcg/hr IV drip × 3–5 d after endoscopic variceal band ligation
  - Transjugular intrahepatic portosystemic shunt is a bridge to transplantation
  - Prophylaxis with propranolol 40 mg PO bid or nadolol 20–40 mg PO daily then titrated to decrease resting pulse 25% (or resting pulse 55–65 bpm)
  - Prophylactic antibiotics × 7 d if acute bleed: decreases the risk of death, SBP, or variceal rebleed
- **Hepatic encephalopathy**
  - Precipitants: GI bleed, medications, high protein intake, infection, or electrolyte disorders
  - Treatments: lactulose 30–45 mL PO tid; titrate to 2–4 loose bowel movements daily
  - Add neomycin 1–3 g PO qid or rifaximin 200 mg PO tid for refractory cases
- **Hepatorenal syndrome:** diagnosis of exclusion; serum creatinine (crt) >1.5 mg/dL or CrCl <40 mL/min and urinary indices mimic prerenal azotemia (UNa <10 mEq/L)
  - No sustained renal improvement after fluid challenge and stopping diuretics
  - **Therapy options:** midodrine 7.5–12.5 mg PO tid **plus** octreotide 100–200 mcg SQ tid; or norepinephrine 0.5–3 mg/hr infusion; duration of treatment is 5–15 d until serum creatinine <1.5 mg/dL
    - Add albumin 1 g/kg IV on day 1, then 20–40 g IV daily
- **Hepatopulmonary syndrome:** dyspnea and deoxygenation accompanying change from a recumbent to a standing position, and usually clubbing is present
  - Diagnosis with radioisotope perfusion lung scan; treatment is liver transplantation
- **Hepatic hydrothorax:** virtually always right-sided pleural effusion +/– ascites
  - 1–2 g/d sodium restriction and diuretics as per large-volume ascites
  - Transjugular intrahepatic portosystemic shunt for diuretic-resistant effusions
  - Therapeutic thoracentesis is acceptable if necessary, but avoid placement of a chest tube

Treatment of Decompensated Cirrhosis

- Orthotopic liver transplant

References: Hepatology 2004;39:1; NEJM 2004;350:1646; BMJ 2003;326:751; Am Fam Physician 2006;74:756; Southern Med J 2006;99:600; J Clin Gastroenterol 2004;38:52; and Clinic Liver Dis 2006;10:371.

Table 9-6 Etiologies of Ascites

High SAAG (≥1.1 g/dL)	Low SAAG (<1.1 g/dL)
• Cirrhotic ascites	• Peritoneal carcinomatosis
• Alcoholic hepatitis	• Peritoneal tuberculosis
• Right-sided congestive heart failure	• Pancreatic ascites
• Multiple liver metastases	• Biliary ascites
• Fulminant hepatic failure	• Nephrotic syndrome
• Budd-Chiari syndrome	• Lupus serositis
• Portal vein thrombosis	• Bowel infarction or obstruction
• Veno-occlusive disease	• Postoperative lymphatic leak
• Fatty liver of pregnancy	

SAAG = serum-ascites albumin gradient; SAAG ≥1.1 g/dL = portal hypertension (97% accuracy).
Adapted from *Hepatology* 2004;39:1.

Evaluation of Ascites
- Diagnostic paracentesis for all new-onset ascites, decompensated liver disease, or for an acute upper gastrointestinal bleed, and send peritoneal fluid for:
  - Protein, albumin, glucose (glc), cell count, lactate dehydrogenase (LDH), and culture (place fluid directly into aerobic/anaerobic blood culture bottles for optimal yield)
  - If SAAG low, consider placing a PPD test and sending fluid for cytology

References: Hepatology 2004;39:1; NEJM 2004;350:1646; South Med J 2006;99:600; and Hepatology 2005;41:1.

ACUTE ABDOMINAL PAIN

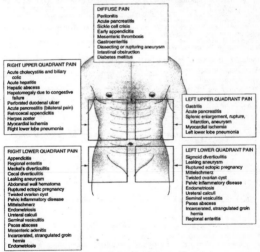

Figure 9-2 Differential Diagnosis of Acute Abdominal Pain
From Wagner DK: Approach to the patient with abdominal pain, Curr Top 1: 3, 1978

HELICOBACTER PYLORI INFECTION

Indications for Testing and Treatment of Helicobacter pylori (H. pylori)
- Peptic ulcer disease (duodenal ulcers or gastric ulcers)
- Ulcer-like dyspepsia
- Atrophic gastritis
- Mucosa-associated lymphoid tissue lymphoma

- Controversial although advised for nonulcer dyspepsia, use of chronic NSAIDs and gastroesophageal reflux disease requiring long-term acid suppression
- Recent resection of gastric cancer
- First-degree relative with gastric cancer
  ➤ Gastric cancer occurs more commonly in patients infected with *H. pylori* compared with age-matched, uninfected counterparts.

Table 9-7 Noninvasive Testing for *H. pylori* Infection

Test	Sensitivity	Specificity	Test for cure
H. pylori stool antigen test*†	89–98%	90–98%	Yes
Urea breath test*	93–100%	98–100%	Yes
H. pylori serum IgG by ELISA	85–95%	89–96%	No
H. pylori urine IgG by ELISA	86–97%	79–96%	No

ELISA = enzyme-linked immunosorbent assay; IgG = immunoglobulins.
* Must be off proton pump inhibitors and H₂-blockers for at least 7–10 d before performing either a urea breath test or an *H. pylori* stool antigen test.
† Test of cure should be done 4 weeks post-therapy and off proton pump inhibitor for ≥1 week.
Adapted from *Best Pract Res Gastroenterol* 2007;21:299–324.

Table 9-8 Treatment Regimens for *H. pylori* Infection

Treatment regimen	Cure rate (%)
PPI* + metronidazole 500 mg bid + clarithromycin 500 mg bid	85%
PPI* + amoxicillin 1000 mg bid + clarithromycin 500 mg bid	78–88%
PPI daily + bismuth subsalicylate 525 mg qid + metronidazole 500 mg tid + tetracycline 500 mg qid	83–95%
bismuth subsalicylate† 525 mg qid + metronidazole 250 mg qid + tetracycline 500 mg qid + (H₂-blocker‡ **or** PPI*) × 14 d	68–95%

* PPI = proton pump inhibitor: oral omeprazole 20 mg bid, lansoprazole 30 mg bid, esomeprazole 40 mg daily, pantoprazole 40 mg bid, or rabeprazole 20 mg bid.
† Bismuth subsalicylate = Pepto Bismol.
‡ H₂-blocker: cimetidine 400 mg bid, famotidine 20 mg bid, nizatidine 150 mg bid, or ranitidine 150 mg bid.
U.S. guidelines for PPI-based triple therapy regimens recommend a 10-d course, and European guidelines suggest that 7 d of therapy is equivalent to 10 d of therapy. Quadruple therapy regimens require a 14-d course.
PPI or H₂-blocker therapy generally continues for at least 2 weeks beyond antibiotic treatment.
Adapted from *Best Pract Res Gastroenterol* 2007;21:299–324.

- Successful *H. pylori* eradication reduces 1-year rate of duodenal ulcer recurrence from 80% to 5% and reduces the rate of gastric ulcer recurrence from 60% to 5%.

Indications for Esophagogastroduodenoscopy
- New-onset dyspepsia if ≥50 yr or associated gastrointestinal bleed
- Alarm signs: unintentional weight loss, anemia, early satiety, or dysphagia
- Dyspepsia or persistent reflux symptoms refractory to appropriate medical therapy
- Dyspepsia that recurs within 3 months of a complete 2-month treatment course for ulcer-like dyspepsia

References: Ann Intern Med *2002*;136:280–287; NEJM *2002*;347:1175–1186; NEJM *2001*;345:784–789; Best Pract Res Gastroenterol *2007*;21:299–324; and Clin Microbiol Rev *2007*;20:280–322.

ACUTE PANCREATITIS

Etiologies
- Gallstones; alcohol; pancreatic divisum; hypertriglyceridemia (TG >1000 mg/dL); severe hypercalcemia; abdominal trauma; post-ERCP; hereditary pancreatitis;

autoimmune (elevated ANA and serum IgG subclass 4); scorpion bite; medications (ACEIs, azathioprine, L-asparaginase, contrast media, didanosine, estrogens, ethacrynic acid, furosemide, glucocorticoids, 6-mercaptopurine, mesalamine, metronidazole, octreotide, opioids, pentamidine, rifampin, stavudine, sulfasalazine, sulindac, tetracycline, thiazides, trimethoprim/sulfamethoxazole, valproic acid, and vinca alkaloids); or idiopathic

Clinical Presentation
• Constant epigastric abdominal pain radiating to back with nausea and vomiting

Diagnostic Studies
• Serum amylase and lipase (usually elevated more than 3 × upper limit of normal)
• Labs: CBCD, chemistry panel, LDH, triglycerides, and oximetry (ABG if hypoxic)
  ➢ ALT level >3 × normal has a 95% likelihood of gallstone pancreatitis
• CXR
• Abdominal ultrasound indicated if gallstone pancreatitis a possibility
• Dynamic CT scan of abdomen with IV/PO contrast using pancreatic protocol if:
  ➢ Hemodynamic instability; or severe acute pancreatitis with persistent SIRS at 72 hr
• Fine needle aspirate of necrotic pancreas for fevers >72–96 hr to rule out infection

Indicators of Severe Acute Pancreatitis (SAP)
• SBP <90 mmHg; PaO2 <60 mmHg; creatinine >2 mg/dL, GI bleed >500 mL/d, or DIC

Table 9-9 Ranson's Criteria

Ranson's criteria		Prognosis	
On admission	At 48 hr	# of criteria	Mortality
Age >55 yr (age >70 yr)	Hct decrease >10% (same)	≤2	<5%
WBC >16K/mm³ (>18K/mm³)	BUN increase >5 mg/dL (>2)	3–4	15–20%
Glucose >200 mg/dL (>220)	Base deficit >4 mEq/L (>6)	5–6	40%
AST (SGOT) >250 units/L (>400)	Calcium <8 mEq/L (same)	≥7	>99%
LDH >350 units/L (>400)	PaO2 <60 mmHg (omitted)		
	Fluid sequestration >6 L (>4 L)		

Criteria for alcoholic (nongallstone) acute pancreatitis listed first; criteria for gallstone pancreatitis in parentheses.
Adapted from *Surg Gynecol Obstet* 1974;139:69 and *Ann Surg* 1979;189:654.

Table 9-10 CT Severity Index

CT grade	Description	Points	Necrosis	Points	Total points	Mortality
A	Normal pancreas	0	<30%	2	0–3	3%
B	Enlarged pancreas; no inflammation	1	30–50%	4	4–6	6%
C	Pancreatic or peripancreatic inflammation	2	>50%	6	7–10	17%
D	Single peripancreatic fluid collection	3				
E	≥2 peripancreatic fluid collections; or gas in pancreas or retroperitoneum	4				

Adapted from *Radiology* 1990;174:331.

- Peripancreatic fluid collection, pancreatic necrosis, pseudocyst, or abscess
- SAP also if APACHE II score ≥8; Ranson's score ≥3; or CT severity index ≥7
- Poor prognostic factors: obesity (BMI >30 kg/m²) and CRP ≥15 mg/dL at 48 hr

Treatment
- NPO; aggressive IV fluid resuscitation (≥5 L/d × 2–4 d) to maintain urine output ≥0.5 mL/kg/hr
- Pain control with IV opioids: morphine or dilaudid preferred over meperidine
- Start enteral feeds if SAP >5 d; nasojejunal elemental feeds probably safer than gastric feeds
- Early ERCP with sphincterotomy ≤72 hr of symptom onset for gallstone SAP with bilirubin >1.2 mg/dL and common bile duct ≥8 mm, or if biliary sepsis present
  ➢ Cholecystectomy once pancreatitis resolved and prior to discharge
- Insulin infusion to keep glucose 100–180 mg/dL
- Close vigilance for the development of acute kidney injury or respiratory failure in first 7 days
- Empiric antibiotics controversial for necrotizing pancreatitis >30% of pancreas

Managing Complications of Severe Acute Pancreatitis
- Indications for drainage of pancreatic pseudocyst: pain, >6 cm, and duration >6 wk
  ➢ Discourage percutaneous drainage because of the risk of infection or fistula formation
- Pancreatic abscess: CT-guided percutaneous drainage and antibiotics
- Infected pancreatic necrosis: open pancreatic necrosectomy and antibiotics
  ➢ Early surgery for hemodynamic instability; delay surgery ≥14 d if clinically stable
- Marked pancreatic ascites: may need ERCP with pancreatic duct stenting if duct disrupted
- Pancreatic fistulas: treat with octreotide infusions or somatostatin injections

References: Crit Care Med 2004;32:2524; Gastroenterology 2007;132:2022; and NEJM 2006;354:2142.

INFLAMMATORY BOWEL DISEASE

Workup of Colitis
- Stool culture, ova and parasites, C. difficile toxin +/– assay for E. coli 0157:H7
- Small bowel follow-through contrast study to rule out strictures consistent with CD

Medical Treatment of Inflammatory Bowel Disease (IBD)
- Avoid narcotics, anticholinergics, antimotility agents, and NSAIDs in active colitis
- Rule out infectious colitis (especially C. difficile colitis) for any flare of CD or UC
- IBD severity: mild disease is <4 stools/d and normal ESR; moderate disease is 4–6 stools/d and minimal systemic toxicity; severe disease is >6 bloody stools/d and fever, tachycardia, anemia, or an elevated ESR; fulminant disease is >10 bloody stools/d, toxicity, abdominal tenderness and distension, and colonic dilatation on KUB

5-Aminosalicylic Acid Derivatives for Mild–Moderate IBD and Maintenance Therapy
- Oral sulfasalazine 1–1.5 g qid or balsalazide 2.25 g tid for colonic involvement
- Mesalamine formulations: Oral Asacol or Pentasa, Canasa suppositories, and Rowasa enemas
  ➢ Asacol 800–1600 mg PO tid for distal ileum and colon
  ➢ Pentasa 500 mg to 1 g PO qid for small bowel and colonic involvement by Crohn disease

Table 9-11 Differentiating Ulcerative Colitis from Crohn Disease

Features	Ulcerative colitis (UC)	Crohn disease (CD)
Passage of mucus or pus	Common	Rare
Rectal bleeding	Common	Rare
Weight loss and growth failure	Occasionally	Common
Perianal disease and fistulas	Absent	Common
Abdominal mass	Absent	Sometimes in RLQ
Colorectal involvement	Exclusively	Common
Ileal involvement	Absent	Common
Esophagus/duodenum/jejunum	Absent	Infrequent
Bowel obstruction	Rare	Common
Cancer	Common	Occasionally
Extraintestinal manifestations*	Slightly less common	Common
Endoscopic findings		
Friability and pseudopolyps	Common	Occasionally
Cobblestoning and linear ulcers	Absent	Common
Distribution	Continuous in colon	Segmental distribution
Lab and pathological findings		
p-ANCA antibodies	60–80% of patients	10–40%
Saccharomyces cerevisiae Ab	6–14%	50–70% of patients
Transmural inflammation	No	Yes
Distorted crypt architecture	Yes	Uncommon
Granulomas	No	Yes (15–36% on biopsy)

p-ANCA = perinuclear antineutrophil cytoplasmic antibodies; Ab = antibodies.
* Arthralgias/arthritis, erythema nodosum, pyoderma gangrenosum, oral ulcers, episcleritis, uveitis, keratitis, myocarditis, pericarditis, ankylosing spondylitis, sacroiliitis, primary sclerosing cholangitis, autoimmune hemolytic anemia, myelodysplastic syndrome, interstitial lung disease, myelopathy, peripheral neuropathy, or secondary amyloidosis
Adapted from *Lancet* 2007;369:1641 and *J Clin Gastroenterol* 2006;40:467.

> Rowasa enemas 1–4 g PR retained for 8 hr qhs for distal colon and rectum
> Canasa suppository 500 mg PR bid–tid or 10% hydrocortisone foam for proctitis
- Maintenance: PO olsalazine 500 mg bid, sulfasalazine 500 mg qid, or mesalamine 1.6 g/d

Corticosteroids for Moderate–Severe CD and UC
- Prednisone 40–60 mg PO daily for moderate CD and UC until clinical improvement, then wean 5–10 mg weekly until 20 mg/d, then decrease 2.5 mg weekly to minimum effective dose
  > Consider budesonide 9 mg/d × 2–3 wk then taper for recurrent or steroid-dependent CD
- Hydrocortisone 100 mg or budesonide 2–8 mg enemas PR daily for proctitis or distal UC
- Methylprednisolone 30 mg IV q12h or 1 mg/kg IV daily for severe CD or UC along with high-dose mesalamine compounds

Immunomodulating Drugs for Refractory Moderate–Severe CD and UC
- Strict bowel rest, IV fluids, and NGT decompression for fulminant colitis or toxic megacolon

- Azathioprine 2.5 mg/kg PO daily or 6-mercaptopurine 1.5 mg/kg PO daily for control of steroid-dependent or refractory IBD or as maintenance therapy of fistulizing CD
- Methotrexate 25 mg SQ weekly for control of moderate, steroid-dependent CD
- Add cyclosporine 2.5–4 mg/kg/d IV as continuous drip after 5 d steroids for fulminant colitis
  ➤ Severe sepsis or death can complicate management

Biologic Agents as Alternatives to Steroids for Induction Therapy of Severe IBD
- Infliximab 5–10 mg/kg IV dose at 0, 2, and 6 wk for severe, refractory IBD or fistulizing CD
- Adalimumab 160 mg SQ × 1 → 80 mg at wk 2 → 40 mg at wk 4 → then q 2 wk if severe CD

Antibiotics for Fistulizing CD, Perianal Disease, or Pouchitis
- Metronidazole 500 mg PO tid or ciprofloxacin 500 mg PO bid

Conditions with Increased Prevalance in IBD
- Thromboembolism, osteoporosis, *C. difficile* colitis, gallstones, nephrolithiasis, and colon CA
- Colon CA screening with colonoscopy after 8–10 yr of colitis then every 1–2 yr

Indications for Colectomy
- Fulminant colitis or toxic megacolon refractory to maximum IV therapy × 7–10 d, severe GI hemorrhage, GI perforation, or high-grade colonic dysplasia or suspected carcinoma

References: NEJM *2002;347:417*; Am Fam Physician *2003;68:707*; Gastroenterol Clin N Am *2004;32:191*; Am J Gastroenterol *2004;99:1371*; GI Endosc *2006;63:546*; and Lancet *2007;369:1641*.

ESOPHAGEAL DISORDERS

Gastroesophageal Reflux Disease (GERD)
- **Definition:** a condition in which the reflux of stomach fluid causes symptoms
- **Common symptoms:** heartburn, regurgitation, atypical chest pain, or dysphagia
- **Less common symptoms:** odynophagia, subxiphoid pain, nausea, chronic cough, hoarseness, laryngitis, poorly controlled asthma, and dental enamel erosions
- **Esophageal disorders:** esophagitis, stricture, Barrett esophagus, and adenocarcinoma
- **Diagnosis:** clinical diagnosis if symptoms typical and good response to therapy
  ➤ 24-hr esophageal pH probe (off PPI or H₂-blockers × 7 d) if diagnosis is equivocal
  ➤ EGD if odynophagia, dysphagia, GI bleeding, unexplained anemia, unintentional weight loss, and symptoms refractory to medical therapy
- **Treatment**
  ➤ **Foods to avoid:** citrus fruits, tomatoes, onions, carbonated beverages, spicy food, fatty or fried food, caffeinated beverages, chocolate, mint, and all bedtime snacks
  ➤ **Lifestyle changes:** smoking cessation, weight reduction, alcohol only in moderation, avoid tight garments and lying down after meals, raise head of bed 6 inches
  ➤ **Medications:** PPI daily–bid or H₂-blocker bid for symptom control
    ○ Chronic use increases the risk of hip fracture, *C. difficile* colitis, and pneumonia (OR 1.4–2)
  ➤ Nissen fundoplication if symptoms refractory to meds or intolerant of meds
    ○ Risks: significant dysphagia (6%), increased flatulence, inability to belch, and increased bowel symptoms

Dysphagia

- **Diagnosis of motility disorders:** esophageal manometry
- **Diagnosis of structural disorders:** barium swallow or EGD
- **Neuromuscular causes of oropharyngeal dysphagia:** stroke, Parkinson disease, multiple sclerosis, myasthenia gravis, amyotrophic lateral sclerosis, polio, polymyositis, dermatomyositis, or idiopathic upper esophageal sphincter dysfunction
- **Structural causes of oropharyngeal dysphagia:** carcinomas, spinal osteophytes, Zenker diverticula, proximal esophageal webs, or prior surgery/radiation to neck
- **Esophageal motility disorders:** achalasia, diffuse esophageal spasm, scleroderma, reflux-associated dysmotility, and idiopathic ineffective esophageal motility syndrome
- **Structural causes of esophageal dysphagia:** carcinomas, benign strictures, mid or distal rings or webs, vascular compression, or eosinophilic esophagitis with/without stricture
- **Medication-induced esophagitis:** bisphosphonates, tetracyclines, quinidine, iron, NSAIDs, aspirin, and potassium chloride
- **Treatment of strictures:** botox injections and pneumatic dilations
- **Treatment of achalasia:** surgical myotomy and a partial fundoplication for achalasia
- **Hypercontractile disorders:** diltiazem and nitrates; add imipramine for atypical CP

Barrett Esophagus (BE, distal esophageal metaplasia)

- **Treatment:** Proton pump inhibitor bid indefinitely
  - ➤ Consider Nissen fundoplication: younger patients and if symptoms refractory to meds
  - ➤ Antireflux surgery superior to meds for regression of BE, but rate of cancer equal
- **Monitoring:** EGD every 3 yr if no dysplasia; yearly for low-grade dysplasia; every 3 mo for focal high-grade dysplasia vs surgery, endoscopic mucosal resection, or mucosal ablation; may screen more frequently if long-segment BE (>3 cm)
- **Indications for surgery:** multifocal high-grade dysplasia or adenocarcinoma

References: Gastroenterology 2008;135:1383; NEJM 2008;359:1700; J Clin Gastroenterol 2005;39:357; J Clin Gastroenterol 2008;42:652; Ann Surg 2007;246:11; J Fam Prac 2006;55:243; and Drug 2005;65(S1):75.

ACUTE MESENTERIC ISCHEMIA

Etiologies of Small Bowel Ischemia

- **Cardioembolism (50%):** most commonly affects the superior mesenteric artery (SMA)
- **Nonocclusive mesenteric ischemia (25%):** shock, post-MI, low cardiac output, severe aortic insufficiency, sepsis, hemodialysis, vasopressors, or postcardiac or postabdominal surgery
- **Mesenteric vein thrombosis (10%):** hypercoagulable states, abdominal trauma, pregnancy, cancer, low flow states, or portal hypertension
- **Mesenteric artery thrombosis (10%):** SMA affected > inferior mesenteric artery (IMA)
- **Focal small bowel ischemia (5%):** vasculitis, small-vessel embolism, or incarcerated hernias

Clinical Presentation of Small Bowel Ischemia

- Sudden onset of severe, colicky abdominal pain out of proportion to exam; associated with abdominal distension, nausea, vomiting, anorexia; +/− GI bleeding if right colon affected

- "Intestinal angina" (postprandial abdominal pain) suggests chronic mesenteric arterial stenosis
- Exam: abdominal distension with minimal tenderness; peritonitis suggests infarcted bowel

Workup of Suspected Mesenteric Ischemia
- **Lab abnormalities:** leukocytosis +/– elevated levels of amylase, CK, and LDH; elevated lactate is a late finding
- **ECG, cardiac monitoring, and 2-D echocardiogram:** evaluates for cardioembolic event
- **Imaging:** KUB normal in mild cases; severe cases: bowel distension, ileus, "thumbprinting"
  - ➢ **CT scan with PO/IV contrast:** identifies intestinal distension, bowel wall thickening, and mesenteric vein thrombosis; pneumatosis intestinalis is a late finding
  - ➢ **CT angiogram:** more sensitive than CT scan for mesenteric arterial thrombosis/stenosis

Treatment of Mesenteric Ischemia
- NPO with bowel rest, volume resuscitation, and discontinue any contributing medications
- NGT decompression to low intermittent suction for severe ileus with abdominal distension
- Antibiotics indicated for signs of intra-abdominal sepsis or bowel infarction
- Acute heparinization if acute mesenteric arterial/venous thrombosis or cardioembolic event
- Options for refractory mesenteric arterial thrombosis or embolism: catheter-directed thrombolysis; surgical embolectomy; or SMA revascularization for SMA thrombosis
- Consider selective mesenteric arteriography with intra-arterial papaverine infusion for nonocclusive mesenteric ischemia
- Indications for surgery: bowel infarction, perforation, or refractory intra-abdominal sepsis

ISCHEMIC COLITIS

Etiologies
- Shock; acute IMA thrombosis; low cardiac output states; cholesterol emboli; colonic obstruction; hypercoagulable states; vasculitis; aortic, colonic, or cardiac surgery; sickle cell disease; abdominal trauma; aortic dissection; post-MI; or vasoconstrictive meds

Offending Meds
- Alosetron, amphetamines, antihypertensives, cocaine, danazol, estrogens, NSAIDs, oral contraceptive pills, pseudoephedrine, psychotropic drugs, and triptans

Clinical Presentation
- Acute onset of crampy, LLQ abdominal pain, anorexia, nausea, vomiting, an urge to defecate, and often passage of red/maroon stool
  - ➢ Exam: focal LLQ tenderness, distension, and ileus; peritonitis suggests bowel infarction

Diagnostic Studies
- Stool for guaiac testing, culture, +/– C. difficile toxin to rule out infectious colitis
- Abnormal labs: none in mild cases; elevated WBC, LDH, amylase, and lactate (late) in severe cases

- ECG, cardiac monitoring, 2-D echo: finds source of cardioembolism in up to 40% of cases
- Imaging: plain x-rays demonstrate bowel distension +/− air-fluid levels
  > CT scan with PO/IV/rectal contrast demonstrates same findings as in mesenteric ischemia
  > CT angiogram is of limited utility, as arterial thrombosis or embolism is essentially never seen
- Colonoscopy diagnostic modality of choice once patient stable: locates segmental ischemia

Treatment of Ischemic Colitis
- NPO with bowel rest, aggressive IV hydration, and discontinuation of offending meds
- Broad-spectrum antibiotics for moderate–severe cases
- NGT decompression with low intermittent suction for severe ileus and distension
- Indications for surgery: peritonitis, persistent intra-abdominal sepsis, symptomatic colonic strictures, persistent symptoms >2–3 weeks, or chronic protein-losing enteropathy

References: South Med J 2005;98:217.

DIVERTICULITIS

Clinical Presentation
- LLQ abdominal pain, fever, and typically with nausea, vomiting, and constipation
- Exam: LLQ tenderness in mild–moderate cases; peritonitis +/− shock in severe cases

Diagnostic Evaluation
- Abnormal labs: leukocytosis; fecal occult blood positive in 25–30% of cases
- CT scan with PO/IV contrast demonstrates diverticuli and sigmoid wall thickening; complicated cases with free air, pericolic abscess, fistulas, or colonic obstruction
- Flexible sigmoidoscopy indicated 2–6 weeks after resolution to rule out cancer

Treatment
- Mild: clears with ciprofloxacin or trimethoprim-sulfamethoxazole DS AND metronidazole; or amoxicillin-clavulanate; duration of therapy is 7–10 d
- Moderate–severe: NPO with IV hydration; NGT decompression only for severe distension
  > Antibiotics: piperacillin–tazobactam; ciprofloxacin + metronidazole; or ampicillin + gentamicin + metronidazole
- Management of pericolic abscesses: percutaneous vs open drainage if abscess >4 cm
- Urgent surgery for: peritonitis, perforation, uncontrolled sepsis, fistula formation, colonic obstruction, or pericolic abscess not amenable to percutaneous drainage
- Indications for delayed colectomy: ≥2 episodes of acute diverticulitis, presence of colon cancer, and potentially after a single severe episode in patients <50 yr
- Prevention of recurrent disease: possible benefit from mesalamine or rifaximin
  > No proven benefit from fiber supplementation once diverticuli have developed

References: Am J Gastroenterol 2008;103:1550; BMJ 2006;332:271; and J Gastroenterol Hepatol 2007;22:1360.

BOWEL OBSTRUCTION

Causes of Small Bowel Obstruction (SBO)
- Adhesions (50–70%); incarcerated hernia (15–30%); volvulus; cancer; intussusception; Crohn disease; or stricture (radiation or prior anastomosis)

Causes of Large Bowel Obstruction (LBO)
- Cancer, complicated diverticulitis, and volvulus are most common; intussusception, foreign body, ischemic colitis, and strictures are less common
  ➢ Cancer is the most common cause of large bowel obstruction in elderly patients

Clinical Presentation of Bowel Obstruction
- Diffuse, colicky pain with abdominal distension; nausea and vomiting
- No flatus or bowel movements in complete SBO/LBO; these are decreased but present in partial SBO

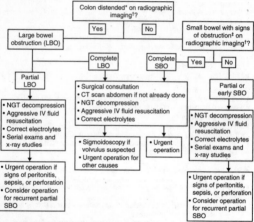

Figure 9-3 Evaluation and Management of Bowel Obstruction
* Cecal distension >9 cm has a high risk of perforation.
† Acute abdominal series or CT scan of abdomen/pelvis with PO/IV contrast.
‡ Distended loops of bowel (>2.5–3 cm), dynamic air-fluid levels, and paucity of large bowel air.

Colonic Pseudo-Obstruction (Ogilvie's Syndrome)
- Occurs in bedbound, hospitalized elderly patients
- **Treatment:** rectal tube or colonoscopic decompression and frequent repositioning
  ➢ Laparotomy and operative decompression if conservative measures unsuccessful or if patient develops worsening abdominal tenderness, fever, or peritonitis

Toxic Megacolon
- Complication of inflammatory bowel disease or *C. difficile* colitis
- Treatment is laparotomy with colectomy and ileostomy, and treatment of underlying condition

References: Am J Surg *2000;180:33;* Gut *2000;47:84;* and J Am Coll Surg *2001;192:422.*

BILIARY TRACT DISORDERS

Acute Cholecystitis

- **Risk factors:** 5 F's are fat, fertile, female, forty, and a positive family history
- **Clinical presentation:** persistent, epigastric or RUQ pain that radiates to the right scapular tip and is associated with nausea and vomiting
  - ➤ Serum bilirubin is usually normal but may increase to 4 mg/dL; jaundice is uncommon
- **Exam:** RUQ tenderness, positive Murphy sign (arrest of inspiration with gallbladder palpation), and fever
- **Diagnostic studies**
  - ➤ Abnormal labs: elevated WBC, alkaline phosphatase, C-reactive protein, and variable rise in liver transaminases and bilirubin
  - ➤ Ultrasound detects gallstones (98% sensitivity), gallbladder wall thickening (≥5 mm), and pericholecystic fluid, and assesses for an ultrasonographic Murphy sign
  - ➤ Hepatobiliary scintigraphy (HIDA scan) with absent gallbladder visualization within 60 min suggests acute cystic duct obstruction (90–97% sensitivity)

Table 9-12 Tokyo Guidelines for the Diagnosis of Acute Cholecystitis

Local symptoms and signs	Systemic signs	Diagnostic imaging
• Murphy sign present	• Fever	• Ultrasound or HIDA scan with abnormal findings*
• RUQ pain or tenderness	• WBC >12.5 K/mm^3	
• RUQ mass palpable	• Elevated C-reactive protein	

Acute cholecystitis if ≥1 local symptom/sign, ≥1 systemic sign, and ≥1 imaging criterion present.
* Abnormal ultrasound if gallstones +/– gallbladder wall thickening or pericholecystic fluid; abnormal hepatic scintigraphy (HIDA scan) if gallbladder not visualized within 60 min.
Adapted from *J Hepatobiliary Pancreat Surg* 2007;14:1.

Table 9-13 Severity Grading and Treatment for Acute Cholecystitis

Grade	Criteria	Treatment recommendations
Mild	Mild inflammation; no organ dysfunction	• Laparoscopic cholecystectomy
Moderate	Presence of ≥1 of following: WBC >18K/mm^3; palpable RUQ mass; duration >72 hr; biliary peritonitis; pericholecystic abscess; hepatic abscess; gangrenous or emphysematous cholecystitis	• Early or delayed cholecystectomy • Antibiotics*
Severe	Presence of ≥1 of following: septic shock; ↓ level of consciousness; acute lung injury; oliguric renal failure; hepatic dysfunction; platelets <100K; or DIC	• Percutaneous cholecystostomy • Antibiotics† • Delayed cholecystectomy

* Mild–moderate infections: cefuroxime or ciprofloxacin and metronidazole; ertapenem; cefotetan; or cefoxitin.
† Severe infections: piperacillin-tazobactam; imipenem-cilastin; meropenem; 3rd-generation cephalosporin or ciprofloxacin; or aztreonam and metronidazole.
Adapted from *J Hepatobiliary Pancreat Surg* 2007;14:78 and *Clin Infect Dis* 2003;37:997.

Acalculous Cholecystitis

- Complicates the course of 1.5% of critically ill patients
- Presents with severe abdominal pain, fever, and minimal abdominal tenderness
- Treatment is with a percutaneous cholecystostomy and empiric antibiotics

Ascending Cholangitis

- **Clinical presentation:** Charcot's triad of fever, jaundice, and RUQ pain in 50–70% of patients
- **Diagnosis:** RUQ ultrasound reveals cholelithiasis; 75% of patients have a dilated common bile duct (CBD); and gallbladder wall thickening
  - ➤ Abnormal labs: leukocytosis (90%); elevated alkaline phosphatase, bilirubin, and variable levels of transaminitis
  - ➤ ERCP is the gold standard study for the diagnosis and treatment of CBD stones
  - ➤ Percutaneous transhepatic cholangiogram (PTHC) and drain placement is an alternative study for diagnosis and treatment if ERCP is unsuccessful or not feasible
- **Treatment:** NPO, IV resuscitation, correct electrolytes and any coagulopathy
  - ➤ Empiric antibiotics: ampicillin + gentamicin; or ciprofloxacin + metronidazole; or monotherapy with either piperacillin–tazobactam, imipenem–cilastin, or meropenem
  - ➤ Duration of antibiotics is 7–10 d
  - ➤ Biliary decompression: ERCP with sphincterotomy or PTHC within 24–48 hr
  - ➤ Delayed cholecystectomy once clinically stable after biliary decompression

Choledocholithiasis

- **Clinical presentation:** RUQ/epigastric pain, jaundice, nausea, and pruritus; up to 50% can present with painless jaundice
- **Diagnostic evaluation:** RUQ ultrasound reveals dilated CBD in 75% of patients
  - ➤ Abnormal labs: elevated alkaline phosphatase, bilirubin, and variable transaminitis
  - ➤ ERCP with sphincterotomy is the diagnostic and therapeutic modality of choice

References: Gastro Endosc Clin N Am 2007;17:289; Curr Gastroenterol Rep 2003;5:302; and NEJM 2008;358:2804.

Section 10
Hematology

TRANSFUSION MEDICINE

Table 10-1 Blood Products and Their Indications

Blood product	Indications for use
Packed red blood cells	Acute blood loss; symptomatic anemia; Hgb <7 g/dL in critical illness; and if Hgb < 10 g/dL and ACS or if SvO_2 <70% in severe sepsis/septic shock
– Leukoreduced	Potential transplant recipients; or prior febrile transfusion reactions
– CMV-negative	Transplant candidates with negative CMV serologies; or patients with AIDS or severe immunodeficiency
– Irradiated	Patients at risk for graft versus host disease (immunosuppression or donor is a first-degree relative)
Platelets	PLT <10K; <50K with active bleeding or requiring a major procedure; if possible, avoid in TTP/HUS, HELLP, HIT, DIC, or APL syndrome
Fresh frozen plasma	Bleeding associated with a coagulopathy; or if INR >2 and/or PTT prolonged preprocedure
Cryoprecipitate	Bleeding associated with vWD, FXIII deficiency, hemophilia; and DIC with fibrinogen <100 mg/dL; risk of viral transmission

APL = antiphospholipid; ACS = acute coronary syndrome.
Adapted from *NEJM* 1999;340:438 and *JAMA* 2003;289:959.

Table 10-2 Infectious Risks of Transfusions

Transmitted infection	Risk	Transmitted infection	Risk
Hepatitis B virus	1:220,000	HTLV-1 or -2	1:600,000
Hepatitis C virus	1:872,000–1,600,000	Bacteremia (platelets)	1:2000–3000
HIV-1	1:1,400,000–1,779,000	Bacteremia (red cells)	1:7000–31,000

Adapted from *NEJM* 1999;340:438; *JAMA* 2003;289:959; and *Transfusion* 2002;42:975.

Massive Transfusion (MT) Protocol
- Defined as the transfusion of 10 or more units of blood within 24 hr
- Complications of MT: hypothermia, thrombocytopenia, coagulopathy, and hypocalcemia
- Minimizing hypothermia: use blood warmers for transfusions
- Platelets: transfuse empirically in pooled platelets to PRBC ratio of 0.8:1; and for PLT <100K
- FFP: transfuse empirically in FFP:PRBC ratio of 2:3
- Cryoprecipitate: indicated if fibrinogen levels less than 100 mg/dL

References: Crit Care Med 2008;36:S325; NEJM 1999;340:438; JAMA 2003;289:959; and Lancet 2003;361:161.

Table 10-3 Transfusion Reactions

Transfusion reaction	Incidence	Signs	Symptoms	Onset of reaction	Treatment & prevention
Acute hemolytic transfusion reaction*	~1 in 250,000	Fever; ↓ HR; hemoglobinuria; renal failure; and DIC	Chills; back or flank pain; SOB; N/V; and dizziness	Within 24 hr of transfusion	Stop transfusion; IV hydration, keep UO >0.5 mg/kg/hr supportive care
Delayed hemolytic transfusion reaction	1 : 1000	Anemia; jaundice; fever; +Coombs; +RBC Ab; ↑ LDH	Usually asymptomatic; possible chills/SOB	Occurs 1–10 d after transfusion	Avoid transfusions with offending antigens
Febrile nonhemolytic reactions	1%	Fever; tachycardia; ↑ blood pressure	Possible chills; rigors; HA; or SOB	During or immediately after transfusion	Stop transfusion; antipyretics; rule out hemolysis
Anaphylactic transfusion reaction*	1 in 20,000–47,000	↑ HR; ↓ BP; ↑ RR; angioedema; stridor; bronchospasm; hypoxia; and urticaria	SOB; chest tightness; nausea; and vomiting	Minutes after starting transfusion	Stop transfusion; IV hydration; secure airway; antihistamines; steroids; epinephrine; check IgA level
Urticarial transfusion reaction	1%	Urticaria; flushing; +/− stridor or wheezing	Pruritus and possibly dyspnea	Minutes after starting transfusion	Stop transfusion; antihistamines; steroids; then may resume transfusion
Transfusion-related purpura†	Very rare	Petechiae, purpura; mucosal bleeding; severe ↓ platelets	Mucosal bleeding; +/− lightheadedness	5–10 d after transfusion	IVIG, steroids; or plasmapheresis; anti-HPA-1a antibody positive
Transfusion-related acute lung injury (TRALI)*	1 : 5000– 10,000	Hypoxia; ↑ RR; fever; ↓ BP; bilat. pulmonary infiltrates; and no CHF	Dyspnea	Usually <2 hr from start of transfusion; never >6 hr	Stop transfusion; mechanical ventilation; avoid diuretics and steroids
Transfusion-related fluid overload	<1%	Hypoxia; ↑ RR; bilat. pulmonary infiltrates	Dyspnea; chest tightness; orthopnea; +/− HA	During or immediately after transfusion	Elevate head of bed; oxygen; and diuretics
Fatal transfusion reaction	1 in 500,000	Severe acute hemolytic reaction or ARDS		Within 6 hr of transfusion	Treatment for problem as above

BP = blood pressure; HR = heart rate; RR = respiratory rate; SOB = shortness of breath; N = nausea; V = vomiting; UO = urine output; RBC = red blood cells; Ab = antibody; HA = headache; PLT = platelets; PRBC = packed red blood cells; HPA-1a = human platelet antigen-1a.
* Send patient's blood to blood bank and send fresh blood for testing.
† Typically occurs in a multiparous woman who develops thrombocytopenia a week after transfusion.
Adapted from *NEJM* 1999;340:438; *JAMA* 2003;289:959; and *Lancet* 2003;361:161.

ANEMIA

Clinical Presentation
- **Symptoms:** fatigue, generalized weakness, exertional dyspnea/lightheadedness, and headache
- **Signs:** pallor, glossitis (iron, folate, B_{12} deficiency), koilonychia (iron deficiency), peripheral neuropathy (B_{12} deficiency), jaundice (hemolysis), splenomegaly (CA, thalassemia, hemolysis)

Peripheral Blood Smear Findings in Different Causes of Anemia
- Basophilic stippling: thalassemias, sideroblastic anemia, and lead poisoning
- Heinz bodies: G6PD deficiency, unstable hemoglobins, and thalassemia major
- Howell-Jolly bodies: sickle cell anemia, and functional or anatomic asplenia
- Hypersegmented neutrophils: megaloblastic anemia (vit B_{12} or folate deficiency); or drugs (azathioprine, hydroxyurea, methotrexate, or zidovudine)
- Nucleated RBCs: chronic hemolysis and any cause of extramedullary hematopoiesis
- Rouleaux formation: monoclonal gammopathies (e.g., multiple myeloma)
- Schistocytes: microangiopathic hemolytic anemia (DIC, TTP/HUS, HELLP syndrome)
- Spherocytes: hereditary spherocytosis, or autoimmune hemolytic anemia
- Spur cells: end-stage cirrhosis
- Stomatocytes: alcoholism and chronic liver disease
- Target cells: chronic liver disease, hemoglobinopathies, or post-splenectomy
- Tear drop cells: myelofibrosis, myelophthisic process (cancer or granulomatous infection in the bone marrow), and megaloblastic anemia
- Toxic granules: sepsis or severe inflammatory states

Evaluation of Normocytic Anemias
- **Labs:** reticulocyte count, serum iron, TIBC, ferritin, B_{12} and homocysteine levels, BUN, creatinine, and an erythropoietin level
  ➤ Homocysteine elevated in B_{12} or folate deficiency
  ➤ Methylmalonic acid elevated in B_{12} deficiency; test if high suspicion and low normal B_{12} level (200–400 pg/mL)
- **Other tests:** urinalysis, CXR, and SPEP with serum immunofixation (for myeloma)
- **Exam:** for signs of occult malignancy (lymphadenopathy, splenomegaly, and stool guaiac test)
- **Anemia of chronic kidney disease:** begins if CrCl <50 mL/min; especially if CrCl ≤ 30
- **Treatment of folate/B_{12} deficiency:** folate 1 mg PO daily; cyanocobalamin 2 mg PO daily

Indications for Bone Marrow Biopsy
- Normocytic or macrocytic anemia of unclear etiology; definitive diagnosis of IDA, sideroblastic anemia, or multiple myeloma; staging/cytogenetic analysis for various cancers

Erythropoietic Agents for Anemia Treatment
- FDA indications: anemia associated with cancer chemotherapy, HIV infection, and CKD
- Off-label uses: myelodysplasia, or ACD due to infection, cancer, or autoimmune diseases
- Supplemental iron indicated if transferrin saturation <20% and serum ferritin <100 mcg/L

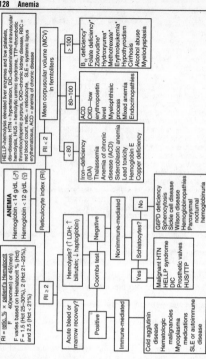

Figure 10-1 Evaluation of Anemia

Iron-deficiency likely if ferritin <30 ng/mL or transferrin saturation ≤8% or ferritin >100. Soluble transferrin receptor (sTfR) can differentiate between ACD and IDA (sTfR/log ferritin >2 = IDA and ratio <1 = ACD). Mentzer ratio (MCV/RBC) >14 suggests iron deficiency or lead toxicity and <12 suggests thalassemia; anemia 2° zidovudine or CKD usually erythropoietin-responsive, bone marrow biopsy indicated for unexplained anemias.

* These anemias usually have MCV >115 femtoliter.

Table 10-4 Evaluation of Microcytic Anemias in Hospitalized Patients

Studies	Iron-deficiency anemia (IDA)	Anemia of chronic disease (ACD)*	Thalassemia	Sideroblastic anemia
Iron (mcg/dL)	<30–50	<30–50	≥50	≥50
TIBC (mcg/dL)	≥250–400	<250	Normal	Normal
Ferritin (mcg/L)	≤100†	>100	>100	>100
Transferrin saturation (Fe/TIBC)	<10%	>10%	≥20%	≥20%
MCV/RBC	≥14	—	≤13	—
RDW	Elevated	Normal	Normal	Normal
PBS findings	Hypochromic	—	• Basophilic stippling • Target cells	Basophilic stippling
sTfR(mg/L)/ log[ferritin(mcg/L)]	>2	<1	—	—
Zinc protoporphyrin (mcg/dL)	>1.24	<1.24	—	—
Hgb electrophoresis	Normal	Normal	Abnormal	Normal
Bone marrow findings	Low iron stores	May be abnormal (infection or CA)	—	Ringed sideroblasts

MCV = mean corpuscular volume; RBC = red blood count; RDW = RBC distribution width; PBS = peripheral blood smear; sTR = soluble transferring receptor.

* Can be from cancer, autoimmune diseases, chronic infections, or chronic inflammatory states.

† Ferritin <50 mcg/L for pts with chronic inflammation, liver disease, or acute illness makes IDA highly likely; ferritin is an acute phase reactant so pts can have IDA with level >100 mcg/L.

Adapted from *Crit Care* 2004;8:S37; *Am Fam Physician* 2000;62:1565; *NEJM* 1999;341:1986; *NEJM* 2005;353:1135; and *NEJM* 2005;352:1011.

> Iron dextran 100 mg slow IVP with epoetin alfa significantly improves Hgb response compared with oral iron supplementation; continue oral iron after Hgb > 10 g/dL
> Target Hgb is ≤12 g/dL; risk of arterial/venous thrombosis, MI/CVA, or tumor progression if Hgb >12 g/dL
- Dose: epoetin alfa 50–100 units/kg SQ 3 × weekly for CKD; 100–300 units/kg IV/SQ 3 × weekly if zidovudine-induced; 40,000 units SQ weekly for chemotherapy-induced anemia
  > Darbepoietin 0.45 mcg/kg IV/SQ every 1–2 wk for CKD; 2.25 mcg/kg SQ weekly or 200 mcg SQ every 2 wk for chemotherapy-induced anemia

Hemolytic Anemias
- **Autoimmune hemolytic anemias (AIHA)**
  > Intravascular hemolysis: markedly elevated LDH; decreased haptoglobin; hemoglobinemia; hemoglobinuria; and positive urine hemosiderin stain
    ○ ABO incompatible transfusion reaction, or paroxysmal nocturnal hemoglobinuria
  > Warm-antibody (IgG): direct Coombs-positive; idiopathic; lymphoproliferative disorders (e.g., CLL); SLE and other autoimmune diseases; HIV; HCV; EBV; and meds

- ○ Meds: cephalosporins, levodopa, methyldopa, NSAIDs, penicillins, penicilla-mine, phenothiazines, phenazopyridine, procainamide, quinidine, rifampin, sulfa drugs, thiazides, and tricyclics (Medication-induced AIHA will have **NO** red blood cell antibodies present.)
    - ○ Warm AIHA treatment: steroids, IVIG, rituximab; splenectomy for refractory cases
  - ➤ Cold-antibody (IgM): idiopathic; monoclonal gammopathies (Waldenstrom macroglobulinemia); CLL; lymphomas; mycoplasma; and infectious mononucleosis
    - ○ Tertiary syphilis and paroxysmal cold hemoglobinuria (IgG-mediated hemolysis)
    - ○ Treatment of cold AIHA: avoidance of cold and consider rituximab or fludarabine
    - ○ Steroids and splenectomy are both ineffective for cold autoimmune hemolytic anemia
- **Nonimmune-mediated hemolytic anemias**
  - ➤ Microangiopathic hemolytic anemias: DIC; HELLP syndrome; TTP/HUS; prosthetic heart valves; and malignant hypertension
    - ○ Treat underlying disease including prompt delivery in HELLP syndrome
    - ○ Urgent plasma exchange for TTP (medical emergency)
  - ➤ G6PD deficiency: hemolysis is precipitated by drugs (aspirin, chloroquine, chlor-amphenicol, dapsone, doxorubicin, metformin, methylene blue, nitrofurantoin, primaquine, pyridium, quinidine, sulfacetamide, sulfamethoxazole, or vitamin C); infection; diabetic ketoacidosis (DKA); or fava beans
  - ➤ Hemoglobinopathies: sickle cell anemia and thalassemias
  - ➤ RBC membrane disorders: hereditary spherocytosis (HS) or paroxysmal nocturnal hemoglobinuria (PNH has an increased risk of venous thromboembolism and aplastic anemia)
    - ○ HS therapy: folate and consider splenectomy for moderate–severe disease
    - ○ PNH diagnosed by peripheral blood flow cytometry (absent CD55 and CD59)
      - ■ Hematology consult: treat with possible stem cell transplant or eculizumab therapy
  - ➤ Infection/toxins: malaria; babesiosis; bartonella; clostridia; or snake/spider envenomations
  - ➤ Hemolytic transfusion reactions: acute or delayed

References: NEJM 1999;340:438; JAMA 2003;289:959; Transfusion 2002;42:975; Lancet 2003;361:161; NEJM 2005;353:1135; NEJM 2005;352:1011; Blood 2004;103:2925; Lancet 2007;369:1502; and Eur J Haematol 2004;72:79.

SICKLE CELL ANEMIA

Diagnosis
- Peripheral blood smear exam is suggestive; hemoglobin electrophoresis is definitive
Management of Complications
- **Vaso-occlusive crises** (bony crises)
  - ➤ Aggressive hydration (3–4 L/d); oxygen; opioids; and NSAIDs
  - ➤ Morphine 4–6 mg IV load then 2–4 mg IV q 5–10 min or hydromorphone 1–2 mg IV load then 0.5–1 mg IV q 5–10 min until pain controlled then initiate an opiate PCA
  - ➤ NSAIDs (unless renal disease): ibuprofen 600 mg PO q6h or ketorolac 30 mg IV q6h (max 5 d)

- **Acute chest syndrome:** acute onset of cough, fever, tachypnea, hypoxia, and alveolar infiltrates; life-threatening complication of sickle cell disease
  - ➤ Treatment: IV hydration, oxygen, antibiotics (e.g., ceftriaxone and azithromycin OR moxifloxacin), exchange transfusion, and frequently necessitates mechanical ventilation
- **Stroke:** in adults, hemorrhagic strokes (especially subarachnoid hemorrhage) > ischemic strokes
  - ➤ Treatment: exchange transfusion followed by maintenance transfusions to decrease the risk of recurrences
- **Avascular necrosis:** commonly affects the femoral head, humeral head, or the acetabulum
  - ➤ Treatment: tissue decompression procedures; or joint replacement
- **Osteomyelitis:** focal pain and fever; occurs at sites of bone necrosis; salmonella > S. aureus
  - ➤ Treatment: 4–6 weeks of IV antibiotics targeting organism identified by bone cultures
- **Skin ulcers:** typically, overlying the lateral malleolus or anterior shins
  - ➤ Local wound care with wet → dry dressings, hydrocolloid dressings, or Unna boots
- **Proliferative retinopathy:** screen annually; laser photocoagulation for neovascularization
- **Renal dysfunction:** hyposthenuria; and papillary necrosis presents as painless hematuria
  - ➤ Treatment of papillary necrosis: IV hydration and urinary alkalinization
- **Cholelithiasis:** present in most adults

Preventative Care

- Immunizations: pneumococcus, haemophilus influenza type b, influenza, and hepatitis B virus
- OCPs, barrier methods, and Depo-medroxyprogesterone acetate are safe contraceptive methods
- Preop care: prophylactic transfusion to Hgb 10 g/dL, generous hydration, supplemental oxygen, and prevent hypothermia prior to general anesthesia
- Consider hydroxyurea 15–35 mg/kg PO daily for ≥3 vaso-occlusive crises/yr or a history of acute chest syndrome
  - ➤ Avoid for severe hypoplastic anemia, leukopenia, thrombocytopenia, or during pregnancy

References: J Emer Med 2007;32:239; Anesthesiology 2004;101:766; NEJM 2008;359:2254; Mayo Clin Proc 2008;83:320; NEJM 1999;340:1021; and NEJM 2008;358:1362.

THROMBOCYTOPENIA

Definition
- Platelet count <150,000 cells/µL (abbreviated as 150K)

Risks of Complications at Different Platelet Counts
- >50K: major surgery safe (except surgery of the brain, spinal cord, or eye—need >100K)
- 20–50K: risk of major bleeding low
- 10–20K: risk of mild–moderate bleeding (low risk for spontaneous hemorrhage)
- <10K: high risk for spontaneous hemorrhage (especially if <5K)

- Consider platelet transfusion if platelets <10K; <20K with active bleeding, infection, or qualitative platelet dysfunction; <50K prior to an invasive procedure or general surgery; <100K prior to neurologic or ophthalmologic surgery
  - ➤ Avoid platelet transfusion in HUS/TTP, antiphospholipid antibody syndrome, HIT, DIC, HELLP syndrome, or severe ITP unless the patient has a severe CNS bleed
  - ➤ 1 unit random donor platelets usually increases platelet count about 10K
  - ➤ 1 unit single donor platelets usually increases platelet count about 50K

Etiologies
- **Pseudothrombocytopenia** (platelet clumping in 0.1% of all blood draws; EDTA-mediated)
- **Decreased platelet production**
  - ➤ Congenital causes (May-Hegglin, Bernard-Soulier, thrombocytopenia with absent radius and Wiskott-Aldrich syndrome and Fanconi syndrome)
  - ➤ Myelodysplasia (>60 yr), lymphoproliferative disorders, or aplastic anemia
  - ➤ Meds/toxins: alcohol, thiazides, estrogens, ganciclovir, and chemotherapy or radiation
  - ➤ Vitamin deficiencies: B_{12} or folate
  - ➤ Infection: sepsis, tuberculosis, measles, HIV, rubella, mumps, parvovirus, varicella virus, hepatitis B virus, hepatitis C virus, and Epstein-Barr virus
- **Immune-mediated platelet destruction** (most common mechanism)
  - ➤ Idiopathic thrombocytopenic purpura (ITP): diagnosis of exclusion with **isolated** thrombocytopenia, normal peripheral blood smear and spleen size
    - ○ Test for *H. pylori* infection and treat for *H. pylori* if present
    - ○ Antiplatelet antibody panel **usually not** useful for diagnosing routine or classic ITP
    - ○ Treatment usually reserved for platelet counts <30K; initial treatment corticosteroids: dexamethasone 40 mg IV daily × 4 d
    - ○ 2nd-line agents: IVIG, $Rh_o(D)$ immune globulin for Rh-positive patient, or splenectomy
    - ○ 3rd-line agents: rituximab, azathioprine, cyclophosphamide, danazol, or vincristine
    - ○ Thrombopoietic agents for refractory ITP: romiplostim or eltrombopag
  - ➤ Evans syndrome: hemolysis, spherocytosis, and positive direct Coombs (DC) test
  - ➤ Meds (common): abciximab, amiodarone, amphotericin B, carbamazepine, cimetidine, clopidogrel, digoxin, fluconazole, heparin, interferon-α, linezolid, penicillins, phenytoin, quinidine, quinine, ranitidine, trimethoprim–sulfamethoxazole, valproic acid, and vancomycin
  - ➤ Meds (less likely): acetaminophen, acyclovir, albendazole, allopurinol, aminosalicylic acid, aspirin, atorvastatin, captopril, cephalosporins, chlorpromazine, chlorpropamide, ciprofloxacin, clarithromycin, colchicine, danazol, deferoxamine, diazepam, eptifibatide, ethambutol, felbamate, furosemide, haloperidol, hydroxychloroquine, inamrinone, indinavir, isoniazid, isotretinoin, itraconazole, levamisole, lithium, mesalamine, minoxidil, nitroglycerin, NSAIDs, octreotide, penicillamine, pentoxifylline, primidone, procainamide, pyrazinamide, rifampin, sirolimus, spironolactone, sulfasalazine, tamoxifen, thiothixene, tirofiban, and ticlodipine
  - ➤ Infection: cytomegalovirus, toxoplasmosis, HIV, Epstein-Barr virus, and *H. pylori*
  - ➤ Miscellaneous: SLE, antiphospholipid antibody syndrome, myelodysplasia, posttransfusion purpura, or type IIB (platelet-type) von Willebrand disease

Table 10-5 Pretest Probability of Heparin-Induced Thrombocytopenia (the 4 "T"s)

Category	2 points	1 point	0 points
Thrombocytopenia	>50% platelet decrease to level ≥20K	30–50% decrease; nadir 10–19K; or >50% decrease postop	<30% decrease; or nadir <10K
Timing of platelet drop	5–10 d; ≤ 1 d if heparin exposure in past 30 d	>10 d; or ≤1 d if heparin exposure in 31–100 d	<4 d and no recent heparin exposure
Thrombosis or skin abnormalities	New thrombosis; skin necrosis; or acute systemic reaction with IV heparin bolus	Progressive or recurrent thrombosis; erythematous skin lesions; or suspected (not proven) thrombosis	None
Other etiologies present	None	Possible	Definite

First day of heparin is day 0. Scoring: high probability = 6–8; intermediate = 4–5; low = 0–3.
Absence of heparin-platelet factor 4 antibodies excludes HIT >95% of the time.
Adapted from *Circulation* 2004;110:e454.

Treatment of Heparin-Induced Thrombocytopenia

- Discontinue heparin/LMWH and start argatroban, lepirudin, or bivalirudin until PLT >150K
- Start warfarin when PLT > 100K and then bridge with warfarin for at least 5 d and until INR 2–3 × 48 hr for treatment of thrombosis
- Fondaparinux is safe for DVT prophylaxis in patients with HIT and platelets >100K
- **Non-immune-mediated platelet destruction** (direct Coombs-negative)
  - ➤ Presence of microangiopathic hemolytic anemia: DIC, HUS/TTP, HELLP syndrome, or malignant hypertension
  - ➤ DIC is associated with sepsis, cancer, trauma, severe pancreatitis, envenomations, hepatic failure, abruptio placentae, or amniotic fluid emboli
  - ➤ Other causes: vasculitis or shearing of platelets on prosthetic heart valves

Table 10-6 DIC Scoring System

Factors	0 points	1 point	2 points	3 points
Platelet count	>100,000	50–100,000	<50,000	—
D-dimer (ng/mL)	≤1000	—	1000–5000	>5000
Fibrinogen (mg/dL)	>100	<100	—	—
Prothrombin time prolongation	<0–3 sec	3–6 sec	>6 sec	—

Overt DIC if score ≥5.
Adapted from *Crit Care Med* 2006;34:314.

- **TTP:** severe deficiency (<5%) of ADAMTS 13 enzyme activity supports idiopathic TTP
  - ➤ Emergent plasmapheresis and glucocorticoids for idiopathic TTP until PLT > 150K
  - ➤ Recurrent TTP or refractory disease: consider corticosteroids, rituximab, or splenectomy
- **Splenic sequestration** (platelets usually >40K)
  - ➤ Portal hypertension, Gaucher disease, lymphoma/leukemias, myelofibrosis, or CHF

- **Gestational** (5% of all pregnancies in late 3rd trimester; platelets usually >70K)
- **Dilutional:** After massive blood transfusions (≥10 units PRBCs)

Workup
- History and exam: assess for splenomegaly or lymphadenopathy and check medication list
- Check peripheral blood smear: platelet clumping, schistocytes, spherocytes, and other cell lines
- Labs: complete blood count with differential and coagulation studies
  - ➢ If schistocytes, confirm hemolysis with markedly elevated LDH and indirect hyperbilirubinemia; check direct Coombs test
  - ➢ If direct Coombs-negative, check DIC panel (positive = DIC; negative = TTP/HUS)
- Consider bone marrow biopsy if etiology unclear; multiple cell lines are abnormal; or patient is >60 yr

References: Mayo Clin Proc 2004;79:504; NEJM 2006;355:809; NEJM 2006;354:1927; NEJM 2007;357:580; NEJM 2006;354:1927; and South Med J 2006;99:490.

PANCYTOPENIA

- **Drug-induced or chemical-induced:** acetazolamide, alcohol, allopurinol, antithyroid drugs, arsenic poisoning, aspirin, benzene, captopril, carbamazepine, systemic chemotherapy, chloramphenicol, chloroquine, chlorpromazine, colchicines, corticosteroids, dapsone, felbamate, furosemide, gold, insecticides, interferon-α, lisinopril, lithium, mebendazole, nizatidine, NSAIDs (butazones, diclofenac, indomethacin, and piroxicam), penicillamine, pentoxifylline, phenobarbital, phenylbutazone, phenothiazines, phenytoin, quinidine, sulfonamides, sulindac, ticlopidine, tolbutamide, thiazides, and toluene
- **Gamma radiation-induced**
- **Bone marrow replacement by cancer:** hematologic or metastatic solid organ malignancies
- **Infections:** bacterial septic shock, or tuberculosis; invasive fungal; brucellosis; babesiosis; HIV; HCV; HBV; non-A, -B, or -C hepatitis virus; CMV, EBV, or parvovirus B19
- **Autoimmune disorders:** systemic lupus erythematosus
- **Hematologic disorders:** aplastic anemia, paroxysmal nocturnal hemoglobinuria, osteopetrosis, myelodysplastic syndromes, and agnogenic myeloid metaplasia with myelofibrosis
- **Megaloblastic syndromes:** vit B_{12} or folate deficiency
- **Miscellaneous:** Gaucher or lipid storage diseases, sarcoidosis, copper deficiency, or Niemann-Pick disease
- **Hypersplenism**

Evaluation of Pancytopenia
- History of recent chemotherapy, radiation therapy, or culprit medication/chemical exposure?
- Exam for occult malignancy, infection, or autoimmune disorder
- Labs: CBCD, chemistry panel, LDH, B_{12} and homocysteine levels, HIV, HCV, and HBV serologies, +/– ANA
- Bone marrow biopsy for unexplained pancytopenia for routine studies, flow cytometry, and cultures for bacteria, acid-fast bacilli, and fungus

References: Lancet 2005;365:1647; Ann Intern Med 2002;136:534; and NEJM 2004; 350:552.

BLEEDING DISORDERS

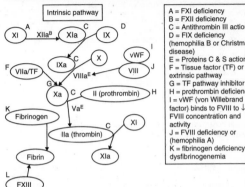

A = FXI deficiency
B = FXII deficiency
C = Antithrombin III action
D = FIX deficiency (hemophilia B or Christmas disease)
E = Proteins C & S action
F = Tissue factor (TF) or extrinsic pathway
G = TF pathway inhibitor
H = prothrombin deficiency
I = vWF (von Willebrand factor) binds to FVIII to ↓ FVIII concentration and activity
J = FVIII deficiency or (hemophilia A)
K = fibrinogen deficiency or dysfibrinogenemia

Figure 10-2 Bleeding Disorders and the Clotting Cascade
Adapted from *Cell* 1988;53:505.

Table 10-7 Coagulation Studies for Various Bleeding Diatheses

Disorder	PTT	PTT with mixing study	PT	Other tests
vWD	↑	NL	NL	RCA + RIPA decreased and low vWD antigen
Hemophilia A	↑	NL	NL	RCA NL and FVIII ↓
Hemophilia B	↑	NL	NL	Decreased FIX
Inhibitors to fibrinogen, II, V, or X or Lupus anticoagulant	↑	↑	↑	Direct inhibitor and lupus anticoagulant testing
Inhibitors to VIII, IX, XI, or XII	↑	↑	NL	Direct inhibitor testing
FV, FVII, or FX deficiency*	↑	NL	↑	Decreased factor levels
FVIII, FIX, FXI, FXII deficiency*	↑	NL	NL	Decreased factor levels
Prothrombin deficiency	↑	NL	↑	Decreased prothrombin
Dysfibrinogenemia	↑	NL	↑	↓ fibrinogen, ↑ TCT
Vitamin K deficiency	↑	NL	↑	Normal TCT
DIC	↑	NL	↑	↓ PLT, ↑ TCT, ↓ fibrinogen, ↑ D-dimer
Severe liver disease	+/– ↑	NL	↑	Abnormal liver panel

vWD = von Willebrand disease; roman numerals refer to specific clotting factors; RCA = ristocetin cofactor activity; RIPA = ristocetin-induced platelet aggregation; PTT = partial thromboplastin time; PT = prothrombin time; TCT = thrombin clotting time; NL = normal; BT = bleeding time; PLT = platelets; Fib = fibrinogen; FSP = fibrin split products; DIC = disseminated intravascular coagulation.
* Single factor levels usually have to decrease to <30% of normal before elevation in PT or PTT is seen.
Adapted from *Haemophilia* 2006;12(S3):68 and *Med Clin N Am* 2001;85:1277.

HYPERCOAGULABLE STATES

Testing Recommendations for Thrombophilia in Venous Thrombosis
- **Strongly thrombophilic states**
  - ➤ Idiopathic VTE <45 yr, recurrent VTE or first-degree relative with VTE <50 yr, a cerebral or visceral vein thrombosis, 1 fetal demise after 10 gestational weeks, or 3 or more unexplained spontaneous abortions occurring at less than 10 weeks gestation
- **Weakly thrombophilic states**
  - ➤ Idiopathic VTE ≥45 yr or occurring during pregnancy, the early postpartum period, or with estrogen therapy and no family history of thrombophilia
- **Timing for testing of hypercoagulable states**
  - ➤ Check all of the lab tests after anticoagulation has been completed and the patient has been off warfarin for at least 2 weeks

Table 10-8 Evaluation of Various Thrombophilic States

Clinical conditions	Tests to consider checking
Strongly thrombophilic states	APC resistance*, prothrombin gene mutation, anticardiolipin antibody, lupus anticoagulant, and levels of plasma homocysteine, antithrombin III, protein C, FVIII activity, and protein S
Weakly thrombophilic states	APC resistance, prothrombin gene mutation by PCR, factor VIII activity, and levels of protein C and protein S
DVT in an unusual site (cerebral, mesenteric, portal, or hepatic veins)	Levels of proteins C and S and antithrombin III, and evaluate for a myeloproliferative disorder (including test for the JAK2 mutation) and for paroxysmal nocturnal hemoglobinuria
Recurrent miscarriages/ stillbirths	Anticardiolipin antibody and lupus anticoagulant

HRT = hormone replacement therapy; APC = activated protein C; PCR = polymerase chain reaction.
* 95% of these cases will be due to a factor V Leiden mutation; check with a factor V Leiden by PCR test.
Adapted from *NEJM* 2001;344:1222.

Suggested Workup for Acquired Hypercoagulable States After VTE Event
- Thorough history (particularly was clot provoked?) and exam (including breast, pelvic, and rectal exam), fecal occult blood testing, urinalysis, complete blood count with peripheral blood smear, chemistry panel, CXR, mammogram (women >40 yr), prostate specific antigen (men >50 yr), and colonoscopy (>50 yr) to evaluate for malignancy
- Urinalysis and serum albumin to screen for nephrotic syndrome
- Inquire about GI symptoms that may represent inflammatory bowel disease
- Examine the patient for orogenital ulcers, uveitis, and skin lesions (Behçet disease)
- Any use of hormonal meds, tamoxifen, raloxifene, erythropoietic agents, or megestrol?

Conditions Associated with Premature Arterial Thrombosis
- Active cancer or myeloproliferative disorders
- Antiphospholipid syndrome
- Hyperhomocysteinemia
- Elevated lipoprotein(a) levels

Screening Asymptomatic Family Members for Genetic Thrombophilia
- No consensus about screening family members of patients with thrombophilia
- Consider screening family members who are contemplating pregnancy or are on treatment with hormonal contraception or hormone replacement therapy
- No role for long-term anticoagulation of asymptomatic patients with inherited thrombophilia and no history of a deep venous thrombosis/pulmonary embolus
  ➤ Avoid screening tests for genetic thrombophilia until after age 15 yr

Indefinite Anticoagulation in High-Risk Patients with Thrombophilia or Unprovoked VTE
- One or 2 unprovoked venous thromboembolic events
- One spontaneous life-threatening thrombotic event
- One spontaneous thrombosis at an unusual site
- Unprovoked VTE and CA, antiphospholipid syndrome, or antithrombin III deficiency

References: Ann Int Med 2001;135:367; Clin Chest Med 2003;24:153; and Lancet Oncol 2005;6:401.

VENOUS THROMBOEMBOLISM

Table 10-9 Risk Factors for Venous Thromboembolic Events (VTE)

Advanced age >50 yr	Recent prolonged travel
Prolonged immobility	Major surgery in last 4 wk
Recent trauma	Inflammatory bowel disease
Previous VTE	Central venous catheter

Medical conditions: severe burns, active cancer, stroke with paresis, inherited thrombophilia, polycythemia, myeloproliferative disorder, obesity, CHF, nephrotic syndrome, inflammatory bowel disease, acute MI, acute respiratory failure, sickle cell disease, paroxysmal nocturnal hemoglobinuria, and pregnancy

Medications: tamoxifen, raloxifene, thalidomide, lenalidomide, darbepoetin, epoetin-α, bevacizumab, hormone replacement therapy, or systemic chemotherapy

Adapted from Arch Intern Med 2002;162:1245 and NEJM 2001;344:1222.

Treatment Options for Deep Venous Thrombosis or Pulmonary Emboli
- Unfractionated heparin 80 units/kg bolus → 18 units/kg/hr titrated to PTT 1.5–2.5 × upper limit of normal
- Enoxaparin 1 mg/kg SQ q12h or 1.5 mg/kg SQ daily (avoid if CrCl <15 mL/min)
  ➤ Dose adjustment required for CrCl 15–30 mL/min
  ➤ Follow anti-FXa levels to adjust dosing for patient weight >150 kg or <45–50 kg
  ➤ For VTE with cancer, use LMWH for ≥6 months; and indefinitely if cancer is still active
- Dalteparin 100 units/kg SQ q12h or 200 units/kg SQ daily
- Tinzaparin 175 units/kg SQ daily
- Fondaparinux 5 mg (<50 kg), 7.5 mg (50–100 kg), or 10 mg (>100 kg) SQ daily
- Overlap warfarin and heparin/fondaparinux ≥5 d and until INR 2–3 for 24 hr
- Early ambulation is recommended for patients with DVT on anticoagulation
- Inferior vena cava filter if anticoagulation is contraindicated or if recurrent pulmonary embolus on therapeutic doses of anticoagulation
- Consider catheter-directed thrombolysis for a massive, limb-threatening ileofemoral DVT with symptoms <14 d, good functional status, and life expectancy ≥1 yr
- Consider IV tPA in a hemodynamically unstable patient with a massive PE

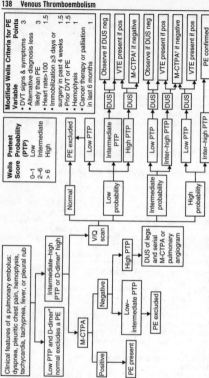

Figure 10-3 Evaluation of Suspected Pulmonary Embolism (PE)
M-CTPA = multidetector CT pulmonary angiogram; DVT = deep venous thrombosis; VTE = venous thromboembolism; DUS = duplex ultrasound;
neg = negative, pos = positive.
* D-dimer ≤500 ng/mL is normal.
† M-CTPA positive, PE present; negative, PE excluded.
Adapted from *Ann Intern Med* 2001;135:98; *JAMA* 2006;295:172; *NEJM* 2006;354:2317; and *Am J Med* 2006;119:1048.

Modified Wells Clinical Prediction Rule for DVT:
Score 1 point for each of the following:
- Active cancer (treatment or palliation in last 6 mo)
- Paralysis, paresis, or recent leg casting
- Bedridden ≥ 3 d or major surgery within 4 wk
- Localized tenderness along deep venous system
- Entire extremity swollen
- Unilateral calf swelling > 3 cm below tibial tuberosity
- Unilateral pitting edema
- Prominent nonvaricose collateral superficial veins
- Score –2 if alternative diagnosis as likely as DVT

Pretest probability	Score
High (75% risk of DVT)	≥ 3
Intermediate (17% risk of DVT)	1–2
Low (3% risk of DVT)	0

Treatment options for proximal DVT
- Unfractionated heparin 80 units/kg bolus → 18 units/kg/hr titrated to PTT
- Enoxaparin 1 mg/kg SQ q12h or 1.5 mg/kg SQ daily
- Dalteparin 100 units/kg SQ q12h or 200 units/kg SQ daily
- Tinzaparin 175 units/kg SQ daily
- Fondaparinux 5 mg (< 50 kg); 7.5 mg (50–100 kg); or 10 mg (> 100 kg) SQ daily
- Concomitant warfarin and overlap with heparin ≥ 5 d and INR 2–3 × 48 hr
- Inferior vena cava filter if warfarin contraindicated or if recurrent DVT on adequate anticoagulation
- Early ambulation on heparin is safe
- Graded thigh-high compression stockings (30–40 mm•Hg at ankles) for 2 yr reduces post-phlebitic syndrome

Clinical suspicion for deep venous thrombosis (DVT)
Clinical features: extremity swelling, pain, warmth, prominent superficial veins, a palpable cord, and/or skin discoloration

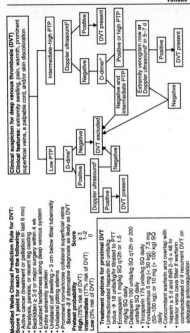

Figure 10-4 Evaluation of Suspected Deep Venous Thrombosis

PTP = pretest probability.
* D-dimer ≤ 500 ng/mL is negative.
† Thrombus seen, noncompressible vessel, and no flow on color flow Doppler imaging.
Note: incidence of occult cancer is 10% with idiopathic VTE; recommend CXR, routine labs, and CT scan of abdomen and pelvis.
Adapted from *Am Fam Physician* 2004;69:2829; *Lancet* 1997;350:1795; *JAMA* 2006;295:199; *Chest* 2008;133(suppl):454; *NEJM* 2004;351:268; and *Ann Intern Med* 2008;149:323.

> ➤ Pulmonary embolectomy is an option for patients at high risk of bleeding
- Graded compression stockings 30–40 mm Hg at the ankle for ≥2 yr after leg DVT

Table 10-10 Duration of Anticoagulation for Venous Thromboembolic Events

Underlying condition or risk factor(s)	Duration
First episode of DVT or PE with reversible risk factors*	3 mo†
First episode of idiopathic VTE or VTE with protein C or S deficiency, elevated FVIII levels, prothrombin gene mutation, hyperhomocysteinemia, or heterozygous factor V Leiden	6 mo†
First episode† of VTE with: active cancer, antiphospholipid syndrome, AT III deficiency, homozygous factor V Leiden, ≥2 thrombophilic conditions **or** for recurrent, idiopathic VTE **or** life-threatening VTE	Indefinite
VTE in pregnancy—anticoagulate until 6 weeks postpartum (avoid warfarin)	
Unprovoked symptomatic distal DVT	3 mo
Symptomatic saphenous or basilic vein thrombosis	4 wk
Infusional superficial thrombophlebitis treated with PO or topical diclofenac	

AT III = antithrombin III.
* Trauma, immobilization, estrogen use, pregnancy, or recent surgery.
† Reevaluate patients after course of anticoagulation with a D-dimer test; recommend continuation of anticoagulation if D-dimer remains elevated (5.4% absolute risk increase of recurrent VTE versus patients with normal D-dimer levels).
Adapted from *Chest* 2008;133:454 and *Ann Intern Med* 2008;149:481.

References: Chest 2008;133(supp):71-109, 454; Circulation 2001;103:2453-2460; and NEJM 2006;355:1780.

Section 11
Infectious Disease

COMMUNITY-ACQUIRED PNEUMONIA

Diagnosis of Community-Acquired Pneumonia (CAP)
- Acute symptoms (cough +/– sputum, dyspnea, fever, +/– pleuritic chest pain)
- Exam: pulmonary rales or rhonchi +/– egophony or tactile fremitus
- CXR or CT scan of the thorax with a pulmonary infiltrate
- Exclude a healthcare-associated pneumonia (HCAP); see pp. 142–143
- Microbiology: *Streptococcus pneumoniae*, *Haemophilus influenzae*, *Moraxella catarrhalis*, *Mycoplasma pneumoniae*, *Chlamydia pneumonia*, and rarely *Legionella pneumophila*

Table 11-1 CURB-65 Score

Confusion (new-onset)	Uremia (BUN > 20 mg/dL)	Respiratory rate ≥30 bpm
Blood pressure (systolic < 90 mmHg, diastolic ≤ 60 mmHg)		Age 65 yr or older

One point for the presence of each item. Recommend ward care if score 2 and ICU care if score ≥ 3.
Adapted from *Thorax* 2003;58:377–382.

Indications for Hospitalization
- PSI class 4–5 (see below); CURB-65 score ≥2; oxygen saturation <90%; unstable comorbid conditions; poor psychosocial situation; failed outpatient therapy; inability to take oral medications; or active substance abuse

Criteria for Severe Community-Acquired Pneumonia
- **Minor criteria:** respiratory rate ≥30; PaO_2/FiO_2 ≤ 250; multilobar infiltrates; acute confusion/disorientation; BUN ≥ 20 mg/dL; leukopenia (WBC < 4000 cells/mm^3); platelets < 100 K cells/mm^3; temperature < 36°C; hypotension resolved with fluid resuscitation; hypoglycemia (in absence of diabetes); acute alcohol intoxication or withdrawal; sodium ≤ 130 mEq/L; lactate > 2 mmol/L; underlying cirrhosis; or asplenia
- **Major criteria:** need for invasive mechanical ventilation; and septic shock
- ICU admission for ≥1 major criteria; ≥3 minor criteria; CURB-65 score ≥3; or PSI class 5
  > Pneumonia Severity Index (PSI) available at www.mdcalc.com/capneumoniarisk

Recommended Diagnostic Studies for Community-Acquired Pneumonia
- Posteroanterior and lateral chest radiograph: examine for infiltrate/effusion
- Pulse oximetry on room air or arterial blood gas (if any concern of adequate ventilation)
- Labs: CBCD, chemistry panel +/– C-reactive protein and HIV test (if age 15–54 yr)
  > Consider urinary antigen tests for Legionella and *S. pneumoniae* if severe CAP
- Sputum culture and Gram stain, and 2 sets of pretreatment blood cultures

Table 11-2 Empiric Antibiotic Therapy for Community-Acquired Pneumonia

Category	Empiric therapy
Non-ICU inpatient	• β-lactam* AND macrolide† OR doxycycline • Respiratory fluoroquinolone‡
ICU patient without pseudomonas risk factors§	• β-lactam* AND azithromycin OR doxycycline • β-lactam* AND respiratory fluoroquinolone‡ • Aztreonam AND respiratory fluoroquinolone‡ (penicillin-allergic patient) • Add vancomycin‖ OR linezolid for MRSA risk factors¶
ICU patient with pseudomonas risk factors§	• Antipseudomonal β-lactam# AND either ciprofloxacin OR levofloxacin • Antipseudomonal β-lactam# AND aminoglycoside AND azithromycin • Aztreonam AND aminoglycoside AND either ciprofloxacin OR levofloxacin (penicillin-allergic pt) • Add vancomycin‖ OR linezolid for MRSA risk factors¶

* Ceftriaxone, cefotaxime, ampicillin-sulbactam, or ertapenem.
† Azithromycin or clarithromycin.
‡ Levofloxacin, moxifloxacin, gatifloxacin, or gemifloxacin.
§ Residence in a long-term care facility, underlying cardiopulmonary disease, recent antibiotics > 7 d or admission for at least 48 hr in the last month, structural lung disease (severe COPD, cystic fibrosis, or bronchiectasis), malnutrition, immunosuppressive illness, or chronic prednisone use > 10 mg/d.
‖ Dose at 15 mg/kg/dose IV q8–12 h with a goal trough of 15–20 mcg/mL (must be renally dosed).
¶ Residence in a long-term care facility, a history of intravenous drug use, post-influenza, sickle cell disease, or a history of MRSA infection.
# Piperacillin/tazobactam, ceftazidime, imipenem, meropenem, or cefepime (infuse each dose over 3 hours).
Note: empiric antibiotics should be initiated within 8 hours of triage into the emergency department
Adapted from *Clin Infect Dis* 2007;44:S27–S72.

Duration of Antibiotics

• Minimum of 5 d and afebrile ≥48 hr with no more than 1 sign of clinical instability: temperature > 37.8°C; HR > 100 bpm; RR > 24 breaths/min; SBP < 90 mmHg; room air SaO_2 < 90% or PaO_2 < 60 mmHg; abnormal mentation; and inability to maintain oral intake
• Longer duration of IV antimicrobials are indicated for bacteremia with *S. aureus*, Burkholderia, fungal pneumonias, and for those with concomitant endocarditis or meningitis

Adjunctive Care for Community-Acquired Pneumonia

• Vaccinate patients for *Streptococcus pneumoniae* and influenza if indicated
• Smoking cessation counseling and pharmacotherapy to assist smoking cessation
• Follow-up CXR in 4–6 weeks to assure resolution of infiltrate

References: Arch Intern Med 2004;164:1807–1811; Am J Med 2004;117:51S-57S; Clin Infect Dis 2007;44:S27–S72; and Clin Infect Dis 2004;39:1783–1790.

HEALTHCARE-ASSOCIATED AND HOSPITAL-ASSOCIATED PNEUMONIAS

Definitions

• Early-onset hospital-acquired pneumonia (HAP): starts 2–4 d after hospitalization
• Late-onset HAP: develops 5 or more d after hospitalization
• Healthcare-associated pneumonia (HCAP) if any of the following risk factors present:
  ➤ Hospitalization for ≥48 hr in last 90 d
  ➤ Resident of a nursing home or long-term care facility

> Received the following in the last 30 d: home infusion therapy or wound care, IV antibiotic therapy, chemotherapy, chronic dialysis; or has attended a hospital-based clinic
> Family member or household contact with a multidrug-resistant pathogen

Risk Factors for Multidrug-Resistant Pathogens
- Antimicrobial therapy within 90 d; late-onset HAP; HCAP; immunosuppressive disease or therapy; and high frequency of antibiotic resistance in community/hospital

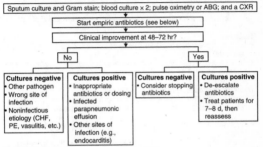

Figure 11-1 Management of Suspected HCAP or HAP
Adapted from *Amer J Resp Crit Care Med* 2005 171:388.

Empiric Antibiotic Therapy
- Early-onset HAP: treat as per CAP without pseudomonas risk factors as in Table 11-2
- Late-onset HAP or HCAP: treat as per ICU patient with CAP and both pseudomonas and MRSA risk factors as in Table 11-2
- De-escalate therapy in 48–72 hr based on culture results and sensitivities
- Duration usually 7–8 d; consider 15 d for nonfermenting GNRs (e.g., pseudomonas)

References: Amer J Resp Crit Care Med 2005;171:388; Clin Infect Dis 2008;46:S296; Clin Infect Dis 2008 46:S378; and Ann Pharmacother 2007;41:235.

URINARY TRACT INFECTIONS: CYSTITIS AND PYELONEPHRITIS

Clinical Presentation
- Cystitis with dysuria, urinary urgency and frequency, and suprapubic pain; fever, nausea, vomiting, and flank pain suggests pyelonephritis
- Microbiology: enterobacteriaceae, enterococcus, and rarely *Staphylococcus saprophyticus*

Diagnosis
- Urinalysis with negative nitrite **and** leukocyte esterase (LE) has a 90% NPV excluding UTI
  > Symptomatic patient with positive nitrite **or** LE: 75% sensitivity; 82% specificity for UTI

- Cystitis if urine culture $\geq 10^5$ colonies/mm^3 or $\geq 10^4$ colonies/mm^3 in catheterized specimen
- Pyelonephritis typically has either full field WBCs in urine or WBC casts

Risk Factors for Cystitis and Pyelonephritis in Women

- Frequent intercourse, obesity, sickle cell disease, urinary calculi, DM or other immunocompromised state, incontinence, pregnancy, neurogenic bladder, and recent instrumentation

Risk Factors for UTI in Men

- Immunocompromised, uncircumcised, age >65 yr, institutionalized, prostatism, neurogenic bladder, recent urinary tract surgery or instrumentation, and engages in anal intercourse

Evaluation

- Urinalysis, urine culture and Gram stain, blood culture × 2, CBCD, and basic metabolic panel
- Renal ultrasound or CT urogram (for stones, renal abscess, or emphysematous pyelonephritis) indicated for pain out of proportion to exam or lack of clinical response within 72 hr

Treatment of Complicated Cystitis or Pyelonephritis

- Urology consultation for emphysematous pyelonephritis, renal or perinephric abscess, or pyelonephritis with an obstructing stone: may need a ureteral stent or nephrostomy tube
- Aggressive IV hydration; analgesia with oral acetaminophen and opioids or IV opioids
- Empiric antibiotics for community-acquired **complicated** cystitis or pyelonephritis
  - ➤ Ceftriaxone, ampicillin and gentamicin, or fluoroquinolone; antibiotic duration is 14 d
  - ➤ Switch to narrowest-spectrum, oral antibiotics based on culture and sensitivity results when clinically improved, afebrile ≥24 hr, and good oral intake
- Empiric antibiotics for nosocomial-complicated UTI (risk of pseudomonas or enterococcus)
  - ➤ Ampicillin and gentamicin; piperacillin–tazobactam; levofloxacin; and imipenem
- Prostatitis:
  - ➤ Age < 35 yr—ceftriaxone 250 mg IM × 1 and doxycycline 100 mg PO bid × 10 d
  - ➤ Age ≥ 35 yr: fluoroquinolone or Bactrim DS for 2–4 wk (acute) or 4–8 wk (chronic)

References: Clin Infect Dis 1999;29:745; J Fam Pract 2007;56:657; Am J Med Sci 2007;333:111; Am J Med 1999;106:327; and Obstet Gynecol 2005;106:1085.

SKIN AND SOFT TISSUE INFECTIONS

Diagnostic Studies

- **Labs:** CBCD, basic metabolic panel, CK, blood cultures, and wound cultures (if pus)
- **Radiology:** plain x-rays for soft tissue gas or foreign body; CT scan for equivocal cases to detect deep abscesses and provide early diagnosis of necrotizing infections

Table 11-3 Management of Skin and Soft Tissue Infections

Infection	Clinical presentation	Microbiology	Preferred treatment	Alternative treatment
Cellulitis (no MRSA risk factors [RFs]: IVDU, purulent drainage, recent hospitalization or antibiotics, hemodialysis, DM, incarceration, contact sports, homosexual men, native Americans, pacific islanders or prior MRSA)	Erythema: warmth, tenderness, and swelling; +/− fever; leukocytosis; and indistinct infection borders.	Streptococcus species Staphylococcus aureus	• Nafcillin • Infections refractory to β-lactam antibiotics ■ Vancomycin	• Cefazolin • Infections refractory to β-lactam antibiotics ■ Linezolid
Cellulitis (MRSA RFs)	Above: purulent drainage	Staphylococcus aureus	• Vancomycin	• Linezolid
Soft tissue infection in neutropenic patients	Red, maculopapular lesions; focal cellulitis; or ecthyma gangrenosum	E. coli, Klebsiella, P. aeruginosa, staphylococci, streptococcus, enterococcus; rarely clostridium	• Piperacillin-tazobactam • Carbapenem	• Nafcillin and aminoglycoside • Cefepime
Erysipelas	Bright red, tender, edematous, and raised border with a sharp demarcation; 80% involves legs; marked lymphatic involvement	Group A streptococcus pyogenes MRSA possible for facial erysipelas	• Penicillin G • Nafcillin Facial erysipelas • Vancomycin	• Cefazolin • Erythromycin (penicillin allergy) Facial erysipelas ■ Linezolid
Uncomplicated cellulitis or infected foot ulcer in diabetic patient	As per cellulitis description above	Streptococcus species Staphylococcus aureus	• Nafcillin	• Cefazolin
Limb-threatening or life-threatening diabetic foot infection	Ulcer with purulent exudate, surrounding cellulitis, tissue necrosis, and gangrene	Streptococcus, Staphylococcus aureus, Enterobacteriaceae, and nonfermenting gram-negative rods	• Vancomycin and piperacillin-tazobactam	• Linezolid and carbapenem • Vanco-, cipro-, and clindamycin
Necrotizing, malodorous DM foot infection	Tissue necrosis, gangrene, crepitus, and foul odor	Polymicrobial with nonfermenting GNRs and anaerobes	• Vancomycin and piperacillin-tazobactam	• Linezolid and carbapenem
Infection after a human or animal bite	Puncture marks; surrounding edema and cellulitis	Oral anaerobes; pasteurella (animals); Eikenella (humans)	• Ampicillin-sulbactam	• Clindamycin and moxifloxacin

Adapted from *Clin Infect Dis* 2004;39:885; *Clin Infect Dis* 2005;41:1373; *NEJM* 2007;357:380; *Ann Int Med* 2009; ITC-2.

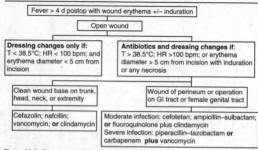

Figure 11-2 Management of Surgical Site Infections
Adapted from *Clin Infect Dis* 2005;41:1373.

Necrotizing Soft Tissue Infections (NSTI)
Risk factors: injection drug use; diabetes; immunosuppression; and obesity
Clinical presentation: tense edema outside the area of erythematous skin; pain disproportionate to appearance; violaceous skin discoloration; blisters/bullae; tissue necrosis; crepitus; cutaneous anesthesia; subcutaneous gas; fever; tachycardia; hypotension; delirium; AKI; and shock
- Progression is usually rapid (especially for group A streptococcus or clostridium species)

Table 11-4 Laboratory Risk Indicator for Necrotizing Fasciitis (LRINEC) Score

Score	C-reactive protein (mg/dL)	WBC (cells/mm³)	Hemoglobin (g/dL)	Sodium (mmol/L)	Creatinine (mg/dL)	Glucose (mg/dL)
0	<15	<15	>13.5	≥135	≤1.6	≤180
1	—	15–25	11–13.5	—	—	>180
2	—	>25	<11	<135	>1.6	—
4	>15	—	—	—	—	—

LRINEC score ≤ 5 is low risk for NF (<50%); score 6–7 = intermediate risk (50–75%); score ≥ 8 = high risk (>75%).
Adapted from *Clin Infect Dis* 2007;44:705.

Treatment: early surgical debridement, source control, and scheduled debridements every 6–24 hr is recommended until no further necrosis or infected tissue is seen
- **Empiric antibiotics**
  - Mixed NSTI
    - Ampicillin + clindamycin + ciprofloxacin or gentamicin **OR**
    - High-dose penicillin G or clindamycin + ciprofloxacin or gentamicin **OR**
    - Monotherapy: carbapenems or piperacillin–tazobactam
    - Add vancomycin, linezolid, or daptomycin to above regimen until MRSA excluded

> Streptococcal NSTI or clostridial myonecrosis: high-dose penicillin G + clindamycin
  ○ Consider hyperbaric oxygen therapy for clostridial myonecrosis
• Consider adjunctive use of drotrecogin-α and IVIG for severe NSTIs associated with severe sepsis or septic shock (especially in streptococcal toxic shock syndrome)

Prognosis: mortality ~ 100% without source control; mortality = 34% with best care

References: Clin Infect Dis *2007;44:705;* Clin Infect Dis *2005;41:1373;* NEJM *2007;357:380;* Clin Infect Dis *2004;39:885;* and Curr Opin Crit Care *2007;13:433.*

MENINGITIS

Table 11-5 Typical Cerebrospinal Fluid (CSF) Parameters

	Normal	Bacterial	Viral	Fungal	Tb	Abscess
WBC/mL	0–5	>1000*	<1000	100–500	100–500	10–1000
%PMN	0–15	>80*	<50	<50	<50	<50
%lymph	>50	<50	>50	>80	↑ monos	variable
Glucose[†]	45–60	<40	45–65	30–45	30–45	45–60
Ratio[‡]	≥ 0.6	≤0.4	45–65	<0.4	<0.4	0.6
Protein[§]	15–45	150–1000	50–100	100–500	100–500	>50
Pressure[∥]	6–20	20–50	variable	>20	>20	variable

WBC = white blood cells.
* Early meningitis may have lower numbers; † mg/dL; ‡ CSF/blood glucose ratio;
§ mg/dL; ∥ Opening pressure in cm H$_2$O.
Adapted from *Emer Med Rep* 1998;19:94 and *JAMA* 2006;296:2012.

General Guidelines for Meningitis Treatment
• Perform blood cultures and lumbar puncture as quickly as possible
• Start empiric antibiotics +/– adjunctive dexamethasone as soon as lumbar puncture completed or prior to CT scan if this precedes a lumbar puncture
• Adjunctive dexamethasone administered prior to or concurrent with antibiotics
  > 10 mg IV q6h × 4 d for meningitis in adults if the CSF is purulent, CSF Gram stain is positive, or if CSF leukocytes >1000/mm^3
• Little role for rapid bacterial antigen testing or Limulus lysate assays unless high likelihood of bacterial meningitis and patient has been receiving antibiotics
• Repeat CSF analysis if no clinical improvement after 48 hr of antibiotics
• Respiratory isolation × 24 hr indicated for any suspected meningococcal meningitis
• **Duration of IV antibiotics:** 7 d for *N. meningitidis* or *H. influenzae;* 10–14 d for *S. pneumoniae;* 14–21 d for *Streptococcus agalactiae;* and 21 d for aerobic gram-negative bacilli or *Listeria monocytogenes*

Table 11-6 Indications for CT Scan of Head Prior to Lumbar Puncture

Age ≥ 60 years	Recent neurosurgical operation or procedure	Immunosuppressed state[†]
Seizure in last week		Dysphasia or aphasia
Gaze or facial palsy	Cognitive impairment*	Focal neurologic deficits
Papilledema	Altered level of consciousness	Abnormal visual fields

* Inability to answer 2 consecutive questions or follow 2 consecutive commands.
† HIV infection, chronic steroids, or post-transplantation.
Adapted from *JAMA* 2006;296:2012.

Cerebrospinal Fluid Tests to Identify Adult Bacterial Versus Aseptic Meningitis

- Individual predictors of bacterial meningitis: CSF glucose <34 mg/dL, CSF/blood glucose <0.23, CSF protein >220 mg/dL, CSF with >1000 leukocytes/mm³, CSF neutrophils >1180/ mm³, or CSF lactate ≥31.5 mg/dL.
- Serum C-reactive protein <1 mg/L excludes bacterial etiology with 99% accuracy
- CSF lactate ≥27 mg/dL predicts bacterial meningitis in postop neurosurgical patients
- Acute meningoencephalitis: start IV acyclovir and send CSF for HSV RNA by PCR; check an MRI of the brain with gadolinium and an EEG to assess for temporal lobe encephalitis
- The workup of aseptic meningitis can be extensive and is beyond the scope of this book.

Table 11-7 Empiric Antibiotic Therapy for Presumed Bacterial Meningitis

Clinical condition/age	Empiric antibiotic therapy
16–50 yr	Vancomycin 30–45 mg/kg/d* plus ceftriaxone 2 g IV q12h
>50 yr or presence of a Listeria risk factor#	Vancomycin 30–45 mg/kg/d* plus ceftriaxone 2 g IV q12h plus ampicillin 2 g IV q4h
Basilar skull fracture	Vancomycin 30–45 mg/kg/d* plus ceftriaxone 2 g IV q12h
Penetrating trauma, CSF shunt, postneurosurgical	Vancomycin 30–45 mg/kg/d* plus cefepime 2 g IV q8h or ceftazidime 2 g IV q8h
Hospital-acquired, neutropenic, or impaired cell-immunity	Ampicillin 2 g IV q4h plus ceftazidime 2 g IV q8h plus vancomycin 30–45 mg/kg/d*

* Maintain serum trough levels 15–20 mcg/mL and give vancomycin as divided doses q6–12 h. # Risk factors for listeria meningitis are alcoholism and an altered immune status.
Adapted from *NEJM* 2006:354:44.

References: Clin Infect Dis *2004;39:1267–1284;* NEJM *2006;354:44–53; and* JAMA *2006;296: 2012–2022.*

INFECTIVE ENDOCARDITIS

Table 11-8 Modified Duke Criteria for the Diagnosis of Infective Endocarditis (IE)

Major criteria	Minor criteria
Positive blood cultures (& no primary focus)	Predisposing heart condition, prior IE, or IVDU
• ≥2 blood cultures positive with typical organisms (strep viridans or bovis, HACEK group, *S. aureus*, or enterococcus)	Temperature > 100.4°F (>38°C)
• Positive blood culture or IgG titer >1:800 for *Coxiella burnetti*	Vascular phenomena: major arterial emboli; septic pulmonary infarcts; mycotic aneurysm; intracranial hemorrhage; conjunctival hemorrhages; and Janeway lesions
Evidence of endocardial involvement	Immunologic: glomerulonephritis; Osler nodes; Roth spots; rheumatoid factor-positive
• Echocardiogram with a pedunculated vegetation; abscess; prosthetic valve dehiscence; new valvular regurgitation	Microbiology: positive blood culture or serologies but does not meet major criteria

Definite IE: 2 major criteria; 1 major and 3 minor criteria; or 5 minor criteria.
Possible IE: 1 major and 1 minor criteria; or 3 minor criteria.
IE rejected: firm alternative diagnosis; resolution of syndrome with antibiotics for < 4 days; no pathologic evidence at surgery or autopsy with antibiotics < 4 d.
Adapted from *Circulation* 2005;111:e394.

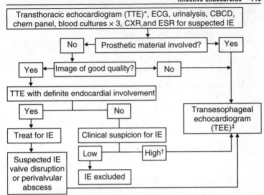

Figure 11-3 Algorithm for Evaluation of Suspected Infective Endocarditis (IE)
* TTE sensitivity = 65%; specificity = 98% for IE.
† High pretest probability for IE if prosthetic valve, congenital heart disease, previous IE, new murmur, new heart failure, sepsis of unknown origin, or other clinical stigmata of endocarditis.
‡ If TEE is negative but clinical suspicion is high, repeat TEE in 3–7 d.
Adapted from *Eur Heart J* 2004;25:267.

Antibiotic Duration for Native Valve (NVE) and Prosthetic Valve Endocarditis (PVE)

- Duration applies to primary therapeutic antibiotic(s); gentamicin used for first 2 weeks only
- NVE: *S. aureus* and enterococcus (6 wk); and HACEK (4 wk)
- NVE: uncomplicated **penicillin-susceptible** (MIC ≤ 0.12 mcg/mL) strep NVE (2 weeks)
- NVE: **penicillin-intermediate** (MIC > 0.12 to ≤0.5 mcg/mL) streptococcus (4 weeks)
- NVE: **penicillin-resistant** (MIC > 0.5 mcg/mL) streptococcus, *Abiotrophia defectiva*, *Granulicatella* sp., and *Gemella* sp. (4–6 weeks)
- PVE: streptococcus (6 weeks); *S. aureus* and enterococcus (6–8 weeks); and HACEK (4 weeks)

Indications for Valve Surgery for IE

- Refractory CHF; persistent vegetation after systemic embolization; increase in vegetation size or persistently positive blood cultures despite appropriate antimicrobial therapy >7 d; acute AI or MR with signs of ventricular failure; valve perforation or rupture; valvular dehiscence, rupture, or fistula; new heart block; perivalvular abscess refractory to antimicrobial therapy; and suspected infection of pacemakers or AICD devices

References: Circulation 2005;111:e394 and Eur Heart J 2004;25:267.

Table 11-9 Antibiotic Therapy for Infective Endocarditis

Organism	Primary IV therapy	Alternative IV therapy
Streptococcus (penicillin-susceptible*) NVE	• Penicillin G[†] + gentamicin[‡] 1 mg/kg q8h × 2 wk	• Ceftriaxone 2 g IV q24h + gentamicin[‡] 1 mg/kg q8h
Streptococcus (penicillin-intermed*) NVE or PVE	• Ceftriaxone 2 g IV q24h + gentamicin[‡] 1 mg/kg q8h	• Vancomycin[§] 30 mg/kg/d + gentamicin[‡] 1 mg/kg q8 h
Streptococcus (penicillin-resistant*) NVE or PVE	• Ampicillin–sulbactam[†] + gentamicin[‡] 1 mg/kg q8h	• Vancomycin[§] 30 mg/kg/d + gentamicin[‡] 1 mg/kg q8h
Methicillin-susceptible *Staph. Aureus* and NVE[‖]	• Nafcillin[†] + gentamicin[‡] 1 mg/kg q8h	• Cefazolin[†] + gentamicin[‡] 1 mg/kg q8h
Methicillin-resistant *Staph. Aureus* and NVE[‖]	• Vancomycin[§]30 mg/kg/d + gentamicin[‡] 1 mg/kg q8h	• Daptomycin 6 mg/kg IV q24h
Enterococcus (penicillin-susceptible*) NVE or PVE	• Ampicillin[†] or penicillin G[†] + gentamicin[‡] 1 mg/kg q8h	• Vancomycin[§] 30 mg/kg/d + gentamicin[‡] 1 mg/kg q8h
Enterococcus (penicillin-resistant*) NVE or PVE	• Ampicillin–sulbactam[†] + gentamicin[‡] 1 mg/kg q8h	• Vancomycin[§] 30 mg/kg/d + gentamicin[‡] 1 mg/kg q8h
HACEK NVE or PVE	• Ceftriaxone 2 g IV q24h	• Ampicillin–sulbactam[†] or ciprofloxacin

NVE = native valve endocarditis.
* Penicillin-susceptible if MIC ≤ 0.12 mcg/mL; intermediate susceptibility if MIC > 0.12 to ≤0.5 mcg/mL; resistant if MIC > 0.5 mcg/mL.
† β-lactam dosing guidelines: penicillin G 3–4 million units IV q4h; nafcillin 2 g IV q4h; ampicillin 2 g IV q4h; cefazolin 2 g IV q6h and ampicillin–sulbactam 3 g IV q6h.
‡ Synergistic gentamicin × **2 weeks** (maintain gentamicin peak 3–4 mcg/mL).
§ Vancomycin given in divided doses q8–12 h aiming for a Vanco trough 15–20 mcg/mL (renal dosing needed).
‖ For prosthetic valve endocarditis (PVE), add rifampin 300 mg IV q8h to regimen.
Note: if possible, avoid systemic anticoagulation during treatment of endocarditis.
Adapted from *Circulation* 2005;111:e394.

OSTEOMYELITIS

Classification of Osteomyelitis
• Acute: evolves in ≤3 weeks
• Chronic: evolves over months to year(s)

Diagnosis of Osteomyelitis
• Chronic osteomyelitis and vertebral osteomyelitis require bone cultures to guide therapy
• **Labs:** WBC is a poor predictor of bone infection
  ➤ ESR and CRP are typically very elevated and more reliable markers of active bone infection
• Imaging procedures
  ➤ X-rays: bone destruction, periosteal elevation, joint space widening after 10–21 d
  ➤ MRI scan: detects early osteomyelitis and soft tissue disease better than CT; appears superior to CT for vertebral osteomyelitis, epidural abscesses, and for DM foot infections
  ➤ Tc-99 m bone scan: uptake with bone infection
    ○ >90% NPV and 80% PPV for bone infection under decubiti

○ Sensitivity 69–100% and specificity 88% if done with gallium scan for acute osteomyelitis

Treatment of Osteomyelitis

- **Acute osteomyelitis:** requires 4–6 weeks IV antibiotics
- **Chronic osteomyelitis:** requires bone debridement, removal of hardware, **and** 4–6 weeks of therapy
- **DM foot ulcers with exposed bone:** requires bone debridement and possible revascularization
  - ➢ PEDIS assessment: Perfusion (arterial inflow), Extent, Depth, Infection, and Sensation
- **Prosthesis-associated osteomyelitis:** generally requires a 2-stage exchange arthroplasty: removal of infected prosthesis; 4–6 weeks IV antibiotics; repeat arthroplasty with antimicrobial-impregnated cement
- **Vertebral osteomyelitis:** 6 weeks optimal duration of antibiotics for vertebral osteomyelitis

Table 11-10 Duration of Antibiotics for Diabetic Foot Osteomyelitis

Bone involvement after debridement	Soft tissue involvement after debridement	Duration of antibiotic therapy
Entire infected bone removed	No infected tissue remains	2–3 d
Entire infected bone removed	Residual soft tissue infection	7–14 d
Viable remnant of infected bone remains	With or without residual soft tissue infection	4–6 weeks
Dead infected bone remains	With or without residual soft tissue infection	≥3 mo (suppressive therapy)

Adapted from *Clin Infect Dis* 2004;39:885–910.

Table 11-11 Antibiotic Treatment for Osteomyelitis

Organism	First-line therapy	Alternative choices
MSSA	• Nafcillin 2 g IV q4–6 h	• Cefazolin 1 g IV q6h • Vancomycin 30–45 mg/kg/d*
MRSA	• Vancomycin IV 30–45 mg/kg/d*	• Linezolid 600 mg IV/PO q12h
Streptococcus	• Penicillin G 4 MU IV q4h	• Clindamycin 600 mg IV q6h • Ceftriaxone 2 g IV daily
Enteric GNRs	• Cipro 400 mg IV q12 h	• Ceftriaxone 2 g IV q24h
Anaerobes	• Clindamycin 600 mg IV q6h	• Ampicillin–sulbactam 3 g IV q6h
Polymicrobial	• Piperacillin–tazobactam 4.5 g IV q6h PLUS vancomycin 30–45 mg/kg/d* or linezolid 600 mg IV/PO q12h	• Imipenem 500 mg IV q6h PLUS vancomycin 30–45 mg/kg/d* or linezolid 600 mg IV/PO q12h

MSSA = methicillin-susceptible *S. aureus*, MRSA = methicillin-resistant *S. Aureus*; GNR = gram-negative rod.
* Dose vancomycin q6–12 h to achieve a serum vancomycin trough level of 15–20 mcg/mL.
Adapted from *NEJM* 1997;336:999 and *Lancet* 2004;364:369.

References: Infect Dis Clin N Am *2005;19:765;* Clin Med *2004;4:510;* Clin Infect Dis *2004;39:885;* Clin Infect Dis *2002;34:1342;* and J Infect *2007;54:539.*

MANAGEMENT OF CATHETER-RELATED BLOODSTREAM INFECTIONS (CRBSI)

Definition
- Bacteremia, fungemia, or clinical sepsis with no other source of infection
- Most common microorganisms recovered in ≥2 blood cultures (1 from peripheral draw and 1 from catheter): staphylococcus, enterococcus, gram-negative bacilli, or candida species
  - ➤ Growth of >15 colony-forming units of same organism from 5-cm segment of catheter tip
- Signs and symptoms of localized infection at the vascular insertion site
- The vascular catheter has been used in the 48 hr preceding a CRBSI

Interventions That Minimize the Risk of a CRBSI
- Good hand hygiene prior to insertion of catheter or accessing catheter ports
- Maximal barrier precautions (sterile gown and gloves, cap, and face mask)
- Chlorhexidine skin antisepsis of insertion area preferred over povidone-iodine
- Optimal site selection (subclavian and internal jugular preferred over femoral vein)
- Daily review of line necessity
- Consider antimicrobial-impregnated catheters if rate of infection >3/1000 line days
- *Avoid* antibiotic ointments to catheter entry sites
- Cover all catheters with a wide transparent sterile dressing

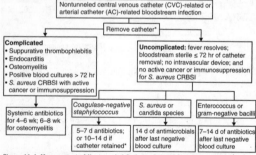

Figure 11-4 Management of Nontunneled Catheter-Related Bloodstream Infections (CRBSI)
* Catheter is removed for all CRBSI, except for *coagulase-negative staphylococcus* when it can be retained and treated with systemic antibiotics **plus** antibiotic lock therapy.
Adapted from *Clin Infect Dis* 2009;49:1–45.

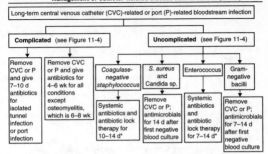

Figure 11-5 Management of Long-term Central Venous Catheter-Related or Port-Related Bloodstream Infections
* CVC or port must be removed for any clinical deterioration or for persisting or relapsing bacteremia.
Adapted from *Clin Infect Dis* 2009;49:1–45.

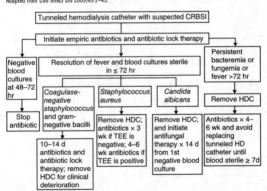

Figure 11-6 Management of Tunneled Hemodialysis Catheter-Related Bloodstream Infections
TEE = transesophageal echocardiogram; HDC = hemodialysis catheter.
Adapted from *Clin Infect Dis* 2009;49:1–45.

SEPTIC ARTHRITIS

Clinical Presentation
- Warm, swollen, exquisitely tender joint; fever; usually monoarticular of hips or knees
- Gonococcal arthritis may be migratory and associated with tenosynovitis or skin rash

Risk Factors
- Age > 80 yr; diabetes; rheumatoid arthritis; recent joint surgery; hip or knee prosthesis; overlying skin infection; HIV-1 infection; fever; and IV drug use

Evaluation
- Labs: WBC > 10,000/mm³; ESR > 30 mm/h; CRP > 10 mg/dL; and send blood cultures × 2
- Arthrocentesis: joint fluid WBC > 25,000/mm³ (usually >50,000/mm³ with ≥90% neutrophils); Gram stain with organisms; +/− fluid for crystal analysis

Treatment
- Arthroscopic joint irrigation and drainage
- Aggressive physical therapy to prevent joint contracture or muscle atrophy
- Antibiotic duration is based on the isolated organism, presence of bone involvement, and the presence or absence of retained hardware

Table 11-12 Empiric Antibiotics for Septic Arthritis Based on Synovial Fluid Gram Stain

Synovial fluid Gram stain	Empiric antibiotic
Gram-positive cocci (no MRSA risk factors)	• Cefazolin 2 g IV q8h
Gram-positive cocci (MRSA risk factors)	• Vancomycin 30 mg/kg/d IV in divided doses
Gram-negative cocci (presumed Neisseria)	• Ceftriaxone 2 g IV q24h
Gram-negative bacilli	• Cefepime 2 g IV q8h or piperacillin–tazobactam 4.5 g IV q6h
No organisms (no MRSA risk factors)	• Cefazolin 2 g IV q8h
No organisms (MRSA risk factors)	• Vanco + piperacillin–tazobactam or cefepime

Adapted from *Infect Dis Clin N Am* 2005;19:799.

References: Infect Dis Clin N Am *2005;19:799;* Am J Emer Med *2007;25:749;* Ann Emerg Med *2008;52:567;* and JAMA *2007;297:1478.*

WORKUP OF FEVER IN THE HOSPITALIZED PATIENT

Definition of Fever
- Temperature: >38°C or 100.4°F

Common Infectious Etiologies of Fever in the Hospitalized Patient
- Hospital-acquired pneumonia
- Catheter-related bloodstream infection
- Urinary tract infections (usually catheter-related)
- *Clostridium difficile*-associated diarrhea
- Surgical site infections (especially if more than 4 d postop)
- Hospital-acquired meningitis (rare in the absence of a neurosurgical procedure)
- Nosocomial endocarditis (beware of pt with a history of IVDU and a new central line)
- Infected decubitus ulcers

Workup of a Nosocomial Fever
- Careful exam for any clinical sources of infection
- **Labs:** CBCD, blood culture × 2, urinalysis and urine culture if ≥5 WBC/hpf, and CXR
- High concern for catheter-related bloodstream infection
  - ➢ Remove line; send tip for semi-quantitative culture (>10⁵ bacteria = CRBSI)
- Three separate stool samples for *Clostridium difficile* toxins A and B if diarrhea
- For new fever and new neurologic findings or delirium, rule out CNS infection
  - ➢ Noncontrast head CT required prior to lumbar puncture for CSF analysis

Noninfectious Causes of Fever
- Drug fever (10% of fevers in hospitalized patients) usually antimicrobials (e.g., β-lactam drugs and amphotericin B), antiepileptic drugs (e.g., barbiturates and phenytoin), antiarrhythmics (e.g., quinidine and procainamide), contrast media, and methyldopa
  - ➢ May take >7 d to resolve after stopping the offending agent
- Malignant hyperthermia
  - ➢ Caused by succinylcholine or inhalational anesthetics (halothane most commonly)
  - ➢ Clinically presents with severe muscle spasms, fever, and elevated creatinine kinase
  - ➢ Usually immediate reaction; may be delayed up to 24 hr in steroid use

Table 11-13 Medical Conditions That Can Cause Fever

Acute myocardial infarction	Jarisch-Herxheimer reaction
Adrenal insufficiency	Pancreatitis
Blood product transfusion	Pulmonary infarction
Cytokine-related fever	Pneumonitis without infection
Dressler syndrome (pericardial injury syndrome)	Stroke
Fat emboli	Substance abuse withdrawal syndromes
Gout	Thyroid storm
Heterotopic ossification	Transplant rejection
Immune reconstitution inflammatory syndrome	Tumor lysis syndrome
Intracranial bleed	Venous thromboembolism

Adapted from *Crit Care Med* 2008;36:1330.

Reference: Crit Care Med *2008;36:1330–1349.*

MANAGEMENT OF INVASIVE FUNGAL INFECTIONS

Table 11-14 Candida Score to Identify ICU Candidates* for Empiric Antifungal Therapy

• Multifocal candida colonization†	• Severe sepsis
• Surgery on ICU admission	• Use of total parenteral nutrition

One point for each risk factor, except for severe sepsis, which receives 2 points. Candida score >2.5 has a sensitivity of 81% and a specificity of 74% for invasive candidiasis.
* Applies only to non-neutropenic pts.
† Surveillance cultures from urine, stomach, and trachea were obtained weekly.
Adapted from *Crit Care Med* 2006;34(3):730–737.

Table 11-15 Recommended Empiric Treatment of Candidal Infections*

Condition	Primary therapy	Alternative therapy
Known or suspected candidemia, nonneutropenic, mod–severe illness or shock	• Echinocandin[†]	• LipAmB 3–5 mg/kg/d • AmB 0.5–1 mg/kg/d • Voriconazole
Suspected candidemia, non-neutropenic, mild illness	• Fluconazole 800 mg IV load then 400 mg/d	• Echinocandin[†]
Known or suspected candidemia, neutropenic	• Echinocandin[†] • LipAmB 3–5 mg/kg/d	• Fluconazole • Voriconazole
Candiduria, asymptomatic	• Remove urinary catheter	• Fluconazole 200–400 mg/d if neutropenic or undergoing a urologic procedure
Candiduria, symptomatic	• Fluconazole 200 mg/d for 2 weeks	• AmB 0.5 mg/kg bladder irrigation daily × 5–7 d
Pyelonephritis	• Fluconazole 200–400 mg/d for 2 weeks	• AmB 0.5–0.7 mg/kg IV daily +/– FC 25 mg/kg qid × 14 d
Chronic disseminated candidiasis	• Fluconazole 400 mg/d • LipAmB 3–5 mg/kg/d	• Echinocandin[†] • AmB 0.5–0.7 mg/kg/d
Osteomyelitis	• Fluconazole 400 mg/d × 6–12 months	• LipAmB 3–5 mg/kg/d or echinocandin[†] × 3 weeks then fluconazole
Septic arthritis	• Fluconazole 400 mg/d × 6 weeks	• LipAmB 3–5 mg/kg/d or echino–candin[†] × 3 weeks then fluconazole
CNS candidiasis	• LipAmB 3–5 mg/kg/d plus FC 25 mg/kg qid × 3 weeks then fluconazole	• Fluconazole 400–800 mg/d until CSF normal and clinical symptoms have resolved
Endocarditis	• LipAmB 3–5 mg/kg/d or AmB 0.6–1 mg/kg/d plus FC 25 mg/kg qid	• Fluconazole 400–800 mg/d as step-down therapy • Valve replacement usually needed
Pericarditis	• LipAmB 3–5 mg/kg/d • Fluconazole 400–800 mg/d	• Echinocandin[†]
Oropharyngeal candidiasis	• Clotrimazole troches • Nystatin swish and swallow	• Fluconazole 100–200 mg/d for mod–severe disease × 7–14 d
Esophageal candidiasis	• Fluconazole 200–400 mg/d	• Echinocandin[†] × 14–21 d
Candida from airway aspirate	• None, as a candida pneumonia is exceedingly rare	

LipAmB = liposomal amphotericin B; AmB = amphotericin B deoxycholate; FC = flucytosine.
* Systemic antifungal may need to be changed based on the eventual candida speciation and sensitivities.
† Caspofungin 70 mg IV load then 50 mg/d; anidulafungin 200 mg IV load then 100 mg/d; or micafungin 100 mg/d.
Adapted from *Clin Infect Dis* 2009;48:503.

Evaluation of Different Forms of Aspergillosis

- Risk factors: immunosuppression, neutropenia, chronic lung disease, and chronic steroid use
- Invasive aspergillosis may present as a necrotizing pneumonia, CNS infection, osteomyelitis, or extension to contiguous intrathoracic structures (e.g., pleura, pericardium, or arteries)
- Cutaneous aspergillosis should be treated as disseminated infection
- Chronic cavitary pulmonary aspergillosis: ≥1 pulmonary cavity with detectable Aspergillus antibodies; usually requires long-term, potentially lifelong, antifungal treatment
- Allergic bronchopulmonary aspergillosis (ABPA): episodic bronchial obstruction; eosinophilia; Aspergillus antibodies present; elevated IgE levels; episodic pulmonary infiltrates; and central bronchiectasis. Can mimic adult-onset asthma.

Table 11-16 Recommended Initial Treatment of Aspergillosis

Condition	Primary therapy	Alternative therapy
Invasive aspergillosis of lungs, sinuses, tracheobronchial tree, CNS, skin, and peritoneum	• Voriconazole 6 mg/kg IV q12h × 2 doses then 4 mg/kg IV q12h → 200 mg PO bid	• LipAmB 3–5 mg/kg/d • Caspo 70 mg × 1 then 50 mg/d • Posaconazole 200 mg PO qid
Endocarditis or pericarditis	• Same medications as above	• Surgical resection required
Osteomyelitis or septic arthritis	• Same medications as above	• Surgical resection of devitalized bone/cartilage required
Endophthalmitis or keratitis	• Intraocular amphotericin B	• Partial vitrectomy often needed
Solitary aspergilloma	• No meds needed, but surgical extirpation needed at times	
Chronic cavitary pulmonary aspergillosis	• Itraconazole 200 mg PO bid • Voriconazole 200 mg PO bid	• LipAmB 3–5 mg/kg/d • Caspo 70 mg × 1 then 50 mg/d
Allergic bronchopulmonary aspergillosis	• Itraconazole 200 mg PO bid • Prednisone 0.5–1 mg/kg/d × 14 d then taper over 3–6 months	• Voriconazole 200 mg PO bid • Posaconazole 400 mg PO bid
Allergic aspergillus sinusitis	• None if mild; itraconazole 200 mg PO bid if mod–severe	

LipAmB = liposomal amphotericin B; Caspo = caspofungin
Adapted from *Clin Infect Dis* 2008;46:327.

Evaluation of Patients with Coccidioidomycosis Infections

- Risk factors for disseminated disease: HIV+; organ transplant patients; use of anti-TNF agents or steroids; lymphoma; DM; and African, Filipino, Asian, Hispanic, or Native American ancestry
- Labs: serum cocci titer; CXR; and bone scan; LP as well if any risk factors for disseminated cocci

Table 11-17 Initial Treatment of Coccidioidomycosis

Condition	Primary therapy	Alternative therapy
Acute pneumonia, mild	• None if uncomplicated in a nonpregnant, immunocompetent patient	
Pneumonia, mod–severe	• Fluconazole 400 mg/d IV or PO • AmB 0.5–1.5 mg/kg/d IV if pregnant	• LipAmB 2–5 mg/kg/d IV • Itraconazole 400–600 mg/d PO
Chronic fibrocavitary pneumonia	• Fluconazole 400–800 mg/d	• AmB 0.5–1.5 mg/kg/d IV until stable then fluconazole
Disseminated, nonmeningeal infection	• Fluconazole 800–1000 mg/d • AmB 0.5–1.5 mg/kg/d IV	• Itraconazole 400–800 mg/d PO
Coccidioidomycosis meningitis	• Fluconazole 800–1200 mg/d • AmB 0.5–1.5 mg/kg/d IV	• Itraconazole 400–600 mg/d PO • Shunt for hydrocephalus

LipAmB = liposomal amphotericin B; AmB = amphotericin B deoxycholate.
Adapted from *Clin Infect Dis* 2005;41:1217 and *Mayo Clin Proc* 2008;83:343.

Table 11-18 Recommended Treatment of Histoplasmosis

Condition	Treatment
Acute (<4 wk) pulmonary histoplasmosis, mild; or pulmonary nodule	• None required
Acute (<4 wk) pulmonary histoplasmosis, mod–severe	• LipAmB 3–5 mg/kg/d **or** AmB 0.7–1 mg/kg/d **or** ABLC 5 mg/kg/d then itraconazole 200 mg PO bid × 12 wk • +/– methylprednisolone 0.5–1 mg/kg/d × 1–2 wk
Chronic (>4 wk) pulmonary histoplasmosis, mild–moderate	• Itraconazole 200 mg PO tid × 3 d then 200 mg bid × 6–12 wk
Chronic cavitary pulmonary histoplasmosis	• Itraconazole 200 mg PO bid for at least 12 months
Pericarditis, mild	• NSAIDs alone
Pericarditis, mod–severe	• Itraconazole 200 mg PO tid × 3 d → bid × 6–12 wk • Prednisone 0.5–1 mg/kg/d tapered over 1–2 wk
Mediastinal lymphadenitis/ granuloma, mild	• NSAIDs or no treatment
Mediastinal lymphadenitis/ granuloma with obstructive or compressive complications	• Prednisone 0.5–1 mg/kg/d tapered over 1–2 wk • Itraconazole 200 mg PO tid × 3 d → bid × 6–12 wk
Mediastinal fibrosis	• Stenting of any obstructed vessels; no antifungals
Disseminated histoplasmosis, mild–mod.	• Itraconazole 200 mg PO bid for at least 12 months
Disseminated histoplasmosis, mod–severe	• LipAmB 3 mg/kg/d **or** AmB 0.7–1 mg/kg/d **or** ABLC 5 mg/kg/d × 1–2 wk then itraconazole 200 mg PO bid for ≥12 months
CNS histoplasmosis	• LipAmB **or** ABLC 5 mg/kg/d × 4–6 wk then itraconazole 200 mg PO bid–tid for ≥12 months

LipAmB = liposomal amphotericin B (Ambisome); ABLC = Abelcet; AmB = amphotericin B deoxycholate.
Adapted from *Clin Infect Dis* 2007;45:807.

Evaluation of Patients with Suspected Histoplasmosis
- Labs: LDH; histoplasma antibody titers (HIV-negative) vs urine histoplasma antigen (HIV-positive)
- Additional studies: CXR; head CT scan and LP if any meningismus or CNS symptoms

INFECTIONS IN HIV-POSITIVE PATIENTS

Table 11-19 Infectious and Noninfectious Complications of HIV Infection

CD4 count	Infectious conditions	Noninfectious conditions
>500	• Acute retroviral syndrome	• Generalized lymphadenopathy
	• Mucucutaneous candidiasis	• Guillain-Barre syndrome
	• Standard bacterial infections	• Medication-induced meningitis
200–500	• Bacterial pneumonia	• Anemia
	• Esophageal candidiasis	• Cervical dysplasia or cancer
	• Herpes zoster virus infections	• Immune thrombocytopenic purpura
	• Localized herpes simplex virus (HSV)*	• Lymphoma (Hodgkin and NHL)
	• Kaposi sarcoma	• Mononeuritis multiplex
	• Oral hairy leukoplakia	• Seborrheic dermatitis
	• Tuberculosis*	
50–200	• Bacillary angiomatosis (Bartonella)	• Cardiomyopathy
	• Disseminated coccidioidomycosis	• Primary CNS lymphoma
	• Cryptococcosis	• HIV-associated dementia
	• Chronic cryptosporidiosis	• HIV-associated wasting syndrome
	• Disseminated HSV*	• Myelopathy
	• Disseminated histoplasmosis	• Peripheral neuropathies
	• Microsporidiosis	• Polyradiculopathy
	• Miliary tuberculosis*	• Immunoblastic lymphoma
	• *Pneumocystis jiroveci* pneumonia*	
	• Progressive multifocal encephalopathy	
	• Toxoplasmosis*	
<50	• Invasive aspergillosis	
	• Disseminated CMV infections	
	• Disseminated Mycobacterium avium complex*	

* Incidence can be decreased with medication prophylaxis.
Adapted from *Infect Dis Clin N Am* 2001;15:433.

CNS Infections
- **Meningitis:** bacterial (including *Listeria monocytogenes*), cryptococcus, viral (HSV, HIV, CMV), *M. tuberculosis*, histoplasmosis, coccidioidomycosis, and lymphomatous meningitis

> **Routine CSF studies:** cell count, glucose, protein, culture and Gram stain, and India ink
> **Other CSF studies:** cocci titer; VDRL; AFB and/or HSV RNA by PCR; and cytology
> **Other studies:** PPD; serum cryptococcal antigen, VDRL and coccidioidomycosis titer; and urine histoplasma antigen

- **Cryptococcal meningitis:** treat with amphotericin B 0.7–1 mg/kg/d or liposomal amphotericin B 6 mg/kg/d **and** flucytosine 25 mg/kg PO q6h × ≥ 2 weeks (watch for cytopenias)
  > Daily lumbar punctures or lumbar drain to keep CSF closing pressure ≤ 20 cmH₂O

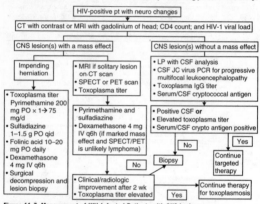

Figure 11-7 Management of HIV-Infected Patients with CNS Lesions
Adapted from *Clin Infect Dis* 2002;34:103; *J Infect* 2000;40:274; and *Neurology* 1997;48:687.

Table 11-20 Chest Radiographic Patterns of Pneumonia in HIV-Positive Patients

CXR pattern	Common pathogens
Focal infiltrate	Bacteria; Tb (especially upper lobes); *P. jiroveci* (uncommon)
Diffuse opacities	*P. jiroveci*; Tb; bacteria; fungal*; cytomegalovirus; Kaposi sarcoma (KS)
Diffuse nodules	Large nodules: KS; small nodules: Tb; *P. jiroveci*; or fungal*
Pneumothorax	*P. jiroveci*
Mediastinal LAD	Tb; nontuberculous mycobacteria; KS; lymphoma; or fungal*
Pleural effusion	Bacteria; Tb; KS; lymphoma; fungal*; cardiomyopathy; or hypoalbuminemia
Cavitation	CD4 > 200: Tb or bacterial; CD4 < 200: *P. jiroveci*; *Pseudomonas aeruginosa*; *Rhodococcus equi*; *Nocardia asteroides*; or fungal*

LAD = lymphadenopathy.
* Fungal includes coccidioidomycosis, blastomycosis, histoplasmosis, and aspergillosis.
Adapted from *Crit Care Med* 2006;34:S245.

GI Infections
- Esophagitis: candida, cytomegalovirus, or herpes simplex virus
- Evaluation of chronic diarrhea
  - Stool for culture, *C. difficile* toxin, ova and parasites, giardia antigen, and special stains for cryptosporidium, isospora, microsporidia, and cyclospora
  - Blood cultures for Mycobacterium avium complex (MAC) (if CD4 < 100)
  - Endoscopy if blood/stool studies unrevealing: small bowel and colon biopsies for MAC, lymphoma, histoplasma, microsporidia, cytomegalovirus, or KS
- Proctitis: herpes simplex virus, cytomegalovirus, chlamydia, or gonococcal infections

Ocular Infections
- Chorioretinitis: commonly CMV; less likely toxoplasma or syphilis; rarely Tb or lymphoma
- CMV retinitis: induction therapy with IV ganciclovir +/– foscarnet or cidofovir
  - Intravitreal ganciclovir implant for maintenance therapy
- Toxoplasma chorioretinitis: treat with pyrimethamine 200 mg PO × 1 then 75 mg/d, sulfadiazine 1–1.5 g PO qid, and folinic acid 20 mg PO 3×/wk
  - Prednisone 1 mg/kg/d tapering over 1–2 wk for vision-threatening disease

References: Lancet *2004;363:1965;* Retina *2005;25:633;* Curr Opin Pulm Med *2005;11:203;* Crit Care Med *2006;34:S245;* Clin Infect Dis *2005;40:480;* and Brit Med Bull *2004;72:99.*

Section 12
Neurology

ACUTE ISCHEMIC STROKE OR TRANSIENT ISCHEMIC ATTACK

- Ischemic strokes account for 85% of all strokes (thrombotic 20%, lacunar 25%, cardioembolic 20%, cryptogenic 30%, or other 5%)
  - ➢ Cryptogenic is most likely embolic and often paradoxical through a PFO
  - ➢ Other causes: hypercoagulable states, dissection, vasculitis, endocarditis, complicated migraine, stimulant drugs, neurosyphilis, paradoxical embolus through a PFO, sickle cell crisis, or a cerebral vein or cerebral sinus thrombosis
  - ➢ Embolic: patients generally experience a sudden onset of maximal deficit
  - ➢ Thrombotic: patients generally have a stuttering or stepwise progression
  - ➢ Paradoxical embolus presents as a sudden neurologic deficit often after a valsalva maneuver
- Hemorrhagic strokes are managed as an acute intracranial hemorrhage (see Figure 5–3, p. 54)

Table 12-1 Clinical Presentation of Acute Ischemic Strokes

Clinical presentation of strokes in carotid distribution	Vascular area
Face and arms affected more than legs, aphasia, hemiparesis, hemianesthesia, contralateral homonymous hemianopsia, and ipsilateral gaze deviation	MCA (dominant)
Face and arms affected more than legs, neglect, hemiparesis, hemianesthesia, contralateral homonymous hemianopsia, and ipsilateral gaze deviation	MCA (nondominant)
Legs are affected more than face and arms, hemiparesis, hemianesthesia, incontinence, personality change, and altered grasp and suck reflexes	ACA
Clinical presentation of strokes in posterior circulation	
Homonymous hemianopsia +/– difficulty with colors	PCA
Ipsilateral cranial nerve palsies and contralateral hemiparesis	Brainstem
Headache, vertigo, vomiting, ataxia, dysarthria, and nystagmus	Cerebellum
Cranial nerve deficits, quadriparesis, somnolence, ophthalmoplegia, dysphonia, dysphagia, and dysarthria	Basilar artery
Vertigo, facial pain, dysphagia, postural instability, hoarseness, ipsilateral Horner syndrome, impaired pain/temperature of face and limb ataxia, and contralateral impaired pain/temperature of limbs	Lateral medullary infarct
Clinical presentation of penetrating artery strokes	
Hemiparesis where legs, arms, and face are equally affected is a pure motor lacunar stroke	Internal capsule (IC)
Hemianesthesia where legs, arms, and face are equally affected is a pure sensory lacunar stroke	Thalamus
Ipsilateral weakness and limb ataxia is an ataxia hemiparesis lacunar stroke	Pons and posterior IC
Clumsy hand-dysarthria lacunar stroke	Pons
Hemiparesis and hemianesthesia where legs, arms, and face are equally affected represents a sensorimotor lacunar stroke	Posterior IC and thalamus

MCA = middle cerebral artery; ACA = anterior cerebral artery; PCA = posterior cerebral artery.

Table 12-2 ABCD* Risk Score for 7-Day Stroke Risk After Transient Ischemic Attack

ABCD Risk Score	7-day stroke risk (%)	95% confidence interval
≤3	0	0
4	2.2	0–6.4%
5	16.3	6–26.7%
6	35.5	18.6–52.3%

* ABCD Risk Score is the total combined points: **A**ge ≥ 60 yr = 1 point; **B**lood pressure elevation at presentation (SBP ≥ 140 mmHg and/or DBP ≥ 90 mmHg) = 1 point; **C**linical features (unilateral weakness = 2 points, speech disturbance without weakness = 1 point, other = 0 points); and **D**uration of symptoms (≥60 min = 2 points, 10–59 minutes = 1 point, < 10 minutes = 0 points).
Adapted from *Lancet* 2005;366:29–36.

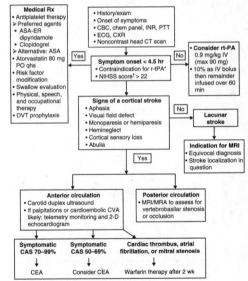

Figure 12-1 Management of Patients with an Ischemic Stroke

ASA = aspirin; ER = extended release; NIHSS = NIH stroke scale; r-tPA = recombinant tPA; CEA = carotid endarterectomy.

* rtPA guidelines for use in acute ischemic stroke available at: www.acep.org/practres.aspx?id = 29936.
† NIHSS available at www.ninds.nih.gov/doctors/NIH_Stroke_Scale.pdf.
Adapted from *Mayo Clin Proc* 2004;79:1071; *NEJM* 2006;355:549; *NEJM* 2008;359:1317; and *Stroke* 2007;38:1655.

Evaluation of Stroke in Young Adults (<50 yr) with Few Vascular Risk Factors
- **Studies:** drug screen, blood cultures, echocardiogram with bubble study, and serum for VDRL, lupus anticoagulant, anticardiolipin antibody, lipoprotein(a) level, homocysteine level, ANA, ESR, ECG, duplex ultrasound of neck (arterial dissection), and sickle cell prep (if patient is African American or of Mediterranean or Southeast Asian descent)

Table 12-3 Secondary Prevention of Ischemic Strokes

Modifiable risk factor	Therapeutic goals/recommendations
Hypertension	BP < 140/90 mmHg (<130/80 for DM or CKD)
Diabetes mellitus (DM)	Hemoglobin A1c ≤ 7%
Sympathomimetic abuse	Abstinence
Smoking	Smoking cessation
Daily alcohol use	Men < 2 drinks; nonpregnant women ≤1 drink
Obesity	Weight loss until waist circumference <35 inches for women and <40 inches for men
Physical inactivity	≥30 min moderate exercise most days
Symptomatic severe CAS	CEA recommended for stenosis 70–99%
Symptomatic moderate CAS	Consider CEA for stenosis 50–69%
Left ventricular thrombus	Warfarin anticoagulation to INR 2.5 (2–3) for 3–12 months
Afib/Aflut	Warfarin anticoagulation to INR 2.5 (range 2–3)
Rheumatic MV disease	Warfarin anticoagulation to INR 2.5 (range 2–3)
Dilated cardiomyopathy	Warfarin anticoagulation or antiplatelet therapy
HMG-CoA Reductase Inhibitors (statins)	Statins beneficial even with normal cholesterol levels and no CAD • Desire LDL <100 mg/dL or <70 mg/dL for very high risk patients* with multiple risk factors
Antiplatelet therapy (ASA, clopidogrel, or ASA-extended-release dipyridamole)	All patients after a noncardioembolic stroke
Prosthetic heart valves	Chronic anticoagulation to INR 2.5 (range 2–3)
Mitral valve prolapse/aortic stenosis	Antiplatelet therapy
Sickle cell disease	Exchange transfusion until Hgb S <30%
Cerebral vein thrombosis	Anticoagulation to INR 2.5 (range 2–3) for 6 mo
Antiphospholipid syndrome	Antiplatelet therapy or chronic anticoagulation to INR 2.5 (range 2–3) if multiple organs involved

CKD = chronic kidney disease; HMG CoA = 3-hydroxy-3-methylglutaryl-CoA; CAD = coronary artery disease; CAS = carotid artery stenosis; CEA = carotid endarterectomy; MV = mitral valve.
* CAD plus diabetes, metabolic syndrome, uncontrolled risk factors, or progressive cardiac ischemia.
Adapted from *Stroke* 2006;37:577–617.

STATUS EPILEPTICUS

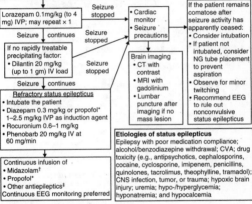

General measures
- Ensure adequate airway; provide respiratory support if necessary
  - Most patients have adequate ventilation if airway is clear
  - Consider placing a nasal trumpet when the seizure has abated
- Position patients so they do not harm themselves
- Check blood sugar: give glucagon 1 mg IM if < 60 and no IV access
  - With IV access, give thiamine 100 mg followed by 1 ampule D_{50} IV
- Assure stable IV access
- Keep core temperature < 40°C
- Rule out reversible causes (see etiologies below)

Lorazepam 0.1 mg/kg (to 4 mg) IVP; may repeat × 1

Seizure continues

If no rapidly treatable precipitating factor:
- Dilantin 20 mg/kg (up to 1 gm) IV load

Seizure continues

Refractory status epilepticus
- Intubate the patient
- Diazepam 0.3 mg/kg or propofol* 1–2.5 mg/kg IVP as induction agent
- Rocuronium 0.6–1 mg/kg
- Phenobarb 20 mg/kg IV at 60 mg/min

Continuous infusion of
- Midazolam†
- Propofol*
- Other antiepileptics‡
Continuous EEG monitoring preferred

Seizure stopped / Seizure stopped / Seizure stopped

- Cardiac monitor
- Seizure precautions

Brain imaging
- CT with contrast
- MRI with gadolinium
- Lumbar puncture after imaging if no mass lesion

If the patient remains comatose after seizure activity has apparently ceased:
- Consider intubation
- If patient not intubated, consider NG tube placement to prevent aspiration
- Observe for minor twitching
- Recommend EEG to rule out nonconvulsive status epilepticus

Etiologies of status epilepticus
Epilepsy with poor medication compliance; alcohol/benzodiazepine withdrawal; CVA; drug toxicity (e.g., antipsychotics, cephalosporins, cocaine, cyclosporine, imipenem, penicillins, quinolones, tacrolimus, theophylline, tramadol); CNS infection, tumor, or trauma; hypoxic brain injury; uremia; hypo-/hyperglycemia; hyponatremia; and hypocalcemia

Figure 12-2 Management of Status Epilepticus
* Propofol 1–2.5 mg/kg load, then 1–4 mg/kg/hr titrated to seizure suppression by EEG; titrate down by 50% over next 12 hr, then off over subsequent 12 hr.
† Midazolam 0.2 mg/kg load, then 0.1–0.2 mg/kg/hr to produce seizure suppression by EEG.
‡ Other options include levetiracetam, high-dose thiopentone or pentobarbital, IV valproate, topiramate, ketamine, isoflurane, lidocaine, and tiagabine.
Adapted from *Chest* 2004;126:582 and *J Neurol Neurosurg Psychiatry* 2008;79:588. Adapted with permission from Mark Lepore, MD.

DEMENTIA

Definition
- Acquired, persistent cognitive impairment that interferes with daily functioning and affects ≥3 cognitive domains: memory, language, visuospatial skills, emotional or personality changes, and poor executive functioning

> Folstein Mini-Mental Status Exam (MMSE) ≤23/30 indicative of dementia
>   ○ Less accurate for age <50 yr, low level of education, or non-Caucasians
>   ○ Other tests: memory impairment score, clock drawing, or word list acquisition

Alzheimer Dementia (50–80% of dementias)
- Gradually progressive deterioration following Functional Assessment Staging (FAST) scale available at www.ec-online.net/Knowledge/articles/alzstages.html
- Additional features: personality changes (extreme passivity to severe hostility); psychotic symptoms (50% with delusions and 25% with hallucinations); mood disorders (40% depressed or anxious); and 30% with Parkinsonian features

Vascular Dementia (10–20% of dementias)
- Stepwise progression of cognitive decline that usually follows a stroke
- Urinary incontinence, gait disturbance, and language impairment are common

Parkinson Disease Dementia (PDD) and Lewy Body Dementia (5–10% of dementias)
- Parkinsonism and graphic; recurrent hallucinations and delusions are common

Frontotemporal Dementia (12–25% of dementias)
- Impaired initiation, goal setting, and planning more than memory loss
- Apathy, disinhibited behavior, conduct problems, poor hygiene, and poor grooming
- Language impairments (logorrhea, echolalia, and palilalia)

Table 12-4 Reversible* Causes of Dementia

B_{12} deficiency	Hypothyroidism	HIV dementia	Neurosyphilis
Normal pressure hydrocephalus (triad of dementia, ataxia, and urinary incontinence)			

* 2% of dementias are fully reversible.

References: NEJM 2004;351:56; Ann Int Med 2003;138:925–937; Neurology 2001;56:1133–1166; JAMA 2004;297:2391–2404; J Psychopharmacol 2006;20:732; and Ann Int Med 2008;148:370–378.

DELIRIUM

The Diagnosis of Delirium Requires the Following 3 Conditions
- Disturbance of consciousness: decreased awareness of environment; poor attention span leading to poor information recall
- Cognitive change: confusion, disorientation, language impairment, +/− psychosis
- Sudden onset, fluctuating severity, disturbed sleep–wake cycle, and transient in nature

Commonly Seen Associated Findings
- Alterations in sleep–wake cycle; mood lability; hallucinations or visual misperceptions

Risk Factors for Delirium
- Advanced age, dementia, medical comorbidities, psychiatric disorder, polypharmacy, depression, social isolation, history of substance abuse, and severity of acute illness

Table 12-5 Etiologies of Delirium

Categories	Specific etiologies (mnemonic = AEIOUMITS)
Alcohol (or illicit drugs)	Alcohol or illicit drug intoxication or withdrawal
Endocrine/Electrolytes/ Environmental	Hyper-/hyponatremia, hypercalcemia, hyper-/ hypothyroidism, Addison disease, Cushing syndrome, and hyper-/hypothermia
Infection/Infarct	Myocardial infarction, hypertensive encephalopathy, hyperviscosity, or any infection
Oxygen (gases)	Hypoxia, hypercarbia, or carbon monoxide poisoning
Uremia	Usually blood urea nitrogen >100 mg/dL
Metabolic/Mental (Psychiatric) or **M**eds (see below)	B_{12} deficiency, Wilson disease, Wernicke and/or Korsakoff syndrome, hepatic encephalopathy, or psychiatric disease (diagnosis of exclusion)
Insulin	Severe hypo-/hyperglycemia
Trauma/Toxins/TTP	Head trauma, toxins (organophosphates, etc.) or thrombotic thrombocytopenic purpura
Seizures, **S**pace-occupying lesion, **S**troke	Stroke, intracranial bleed, brain tumor, hydrocephalus, or seizure
Commonly implicated medications	
Anticholinergics, amiodarone, α-blockers, amantadine, amphotericin B, anticonvulsants, antihistamines, antiparkinsonian meds, aspirin, baclofen, barbiturates, benzodiazepines, β-blockers, bromocriptine, cephalosporins, chlorpromazine, clonidine, colchicine, digoxin, disopyramide, fluoroquinolones, GI antispasmodics, glucocorticoids, histamine receptor$_2$ blockers, levodopa, lithium, metoclopramide, methyldopa, neuroleptics, nifedipine, NSAIDs, opioids, oseltamivir, penicillins, pentamidine, pergolide, pramipexole, procainamide, prochlorperazine, promethazine, quinidine, ropinirole, sedatives, sympathomimetics, theophylline, tricyclic antidepressants, tuberculosis meds, zalcitabine, zidovudine, and zolpidem	

Adapted from *Emer Med Clin N Am* 2000;18:243 and *Am Fam Physician* 1997;55:1773.

Treatment of Delirium
- Detailed history, exam, and lab evaluation for above conditions
- Pharmacologic interventions
  - ➤ Discontinue all nonessential meds and treat underlying condition(s)
  - ➤ Low-dose haloperidol (0.5–2.5 mg IM/IV q0.5–1 h prn for agitation or psychotic symptoms)
  - ➤ Control pain with scheduled analgesics
  - ➤ Minimize use of benzodiazepines
- Nonpharmacologic interventions
  - ➤ Quiet room with familiar objects and family/friends to calm and reorient patient
  - ➤ Maintain adequate hydration and avoid hypoxia
  - ➤ Early mobilization with physical and occupational therapy
  - ➤ Use sensory aids to correct visual and auditory impairments
  - ➤ Maintain consistent caregivers and constantly reorient/reassure patient
  - ➤ Avoid overstimulation and change lighting to cue day and night

References: Emer Med Clin N Am *2000;18:243;* Am Fam Physician *1997;55:1773; and* Chest *2007;132:624.*

WEAKNESS

Causes of Generalized Weakness

- **Electrolytes:** low levels of potassium, phosphate, magnesium, or sodium; or elevated levels of sodium or calcium
- Periodic paralysis (look for hypokalemia or hyperthyroidism)
- Depression
- Medical problems: anemia, chronic ischemic or congestive cardiomyopathy, COPD, adrenal insufficiency, thyroid disorders, anorexia nervosa, cachexia of malignancy, or AIDS

Patterns of Weakness

- Upper motor neuron (UMN): increased tone, hyperreflexia, positive Babinski sign, and spastic
- Lower motor neuron (LMN): hypotonia, hyporeflexia, negative Babinski sign, severe atrophy, fasciculations, fibrillations, and flaccid paralysis
- Myopathic: mild atrophy, proximal weakness, normal DTRs, and negative Babinski sign

Table 12-6 Weakness Syndromes

Defect location	Clinical features	Diagnostic test
Cortex	Contralateral hemiparesis and hemianesthesia and upper motor neuron pattern present	CT/MRI
Internal capsule	"Pure motor" lacunar syndrome and UMN pattern present	CT/MRI
Brainstem	Ipsilateral cranial nerve palsies, contralateral hemiparesis, and UMN pattern present	MRI
Spinal cord lesion	Sensory level, bilateral weakness, and UMN pattern present	Spinal MRI
Brown-Sequard syndrome	Hemiparesis, ipsilateral decreased proprioception, and contralateral decreased pain/temperature	Spinal MRI
Radiculopathy	Back and dermatomal pain/weakness, hyporeflexia	Spinal MRI
Anterior horn cells (polio)	Asymmetric monoparesis, lower motor neuron pattern present, and normal sensation	Clinical
Amyotrophic lateral sclerosis	Any combination of LMN and UMN weakness in bulbar, cervical, thoracic, or lumbosacral innervated muscles	Clinical
Peripheral nerves	Nerve distribution, lower motor neuron pattern present	EMG/NCS
Myopathies	Proximal muscle weakness	EMG and muscle biopsy
PMR	Pain and stiff hip/shoulder girdles, and ESR > 50	Clinical
Rhabdomyolysis	Increased CK and sore muscles	Elevated CK

EMG = electromyogram; NCS = nerve conduction studies; DTR = deep tendon reflexes; ESR = erythrocyte sedimentation rate; CK = creatinine phosphokinase; PMR = polymyalgia rheumatica; MRI = magnetic resonance imaging; LP = lumbar puncture; CT = computed tomography.

Causes of Myopathies

- Alcohol, postviral, polymyositis, dermatomyositis, inclusion body myositis, hyperpara-thyroidism, thyrotoxicosis, myotonic or limb-girdle muscular dystrophies or medications (amiodarone, chloroquine, cimetidine, colchicine, fenofibrate, gemfibrozil, hydroxychloroquine, interferon, lamivudine, leuprolide acetate, methimazole, penicillamine, penicillins, propylthiouracil, statins, steroids, sulfonamides, and zidovudine.

Workup of Weakness

- Is the weakness generalized or does it fit one of the weakness syndromes in Table 12-6?
- **Evaluation of generalized weakness**
  - ➤ Assess for depression or chronic cardiopulmonary disease
  - ➤ Labs: CHEM-7 panel, magnesium, phosphate, calcium, thyroid stimulating hormone (TSH) level, and complete blood count
  - ➤ Cosyntropin stimulation test for any suspicion of adrenal insufficiency
  - ➤ Consider a CXR for adult smokers or those with a chronic cough
- **Evaluation of weakness syndromes**
  - ➤ Start with the diagnostic test of choice as outlined in Table 12-6.
  - ➤ For myopathies or myositis, check an erythrocyte sedimentation rate, creatine kinase, antinuclear antibody test, EMG; consider an open muscle biopsy of the affected muscle for routine pathology and electron microscopy.
- **Evaluation of peripheral neuropathies**
  - ➤ Examine for any medication culprits
  - ➤ Routine labs: CHEM-7 panel, TSH, B_{12} and folate levels, serum protein electrophoresis, and a venereal disease research laboratory (VDRL) test
  - ➤ Additional labs if the history and exam are suggestive: antinuclear antibody, anti-SSA and anti-SSB (Sjogren syndrome A and B) antibodies, serum cryoglobulins, angiotensin-converting enzyme (ACE) level, and HIV test

Guillain-Barré Syndrome (GBS)

- **Clinical presentation:** subacute onset of ascending paralysis, areflexia, or severe hyporeflexia +/− paresthesias/numbness, dysautonomia, and muscle aches
  - ➤ Miller Fisher variant is characterized by the triad of ophthalmoplegia, ataxia, and areflexia
- **Diagnosis:** clinical; CSF with elevated protein and normal WBCs; electromyography and nerve conduction studies confirm the diagnosis; antecedent URI or *C. jejuni* infection in 2/3 of cases
- **Monitoring:** serial forced vital capacity (FVC); consider elective intubation if FVC < 15 mL/kg
- **Treatment:** plasma exchange × 5 sessions or IVIG 0.4 g/kg/d × 5 d are equally efficacious

Myasthenia Gravis Crisis (MGC)

- **Clinical presentation:** ocular, bulbar, or generalized fatigable weakness with diplopia, ptosis, dysphagia, dysarthria, dyspnea, difficulty chewing, +/− proximal limb weakness
- **Diagnosis:** improvement with edrophonium (Tensilon) test; positive α-acetylcholine receptor antibodies
- **Precipitants:** infection, aspiration, surgery, trauma, stress, meds (aminoglycosides, β-blockers, botulinum toxin, calcium channel blockers, cisplatin, clindamycin, colchicines, corticosteroids, diphenhydramine, erythromycin, lithium, penicillamine,

Table 12-7 Spinal Root and Peripheral Nerve Lesions

Root	Disc	Muscles	Weakness	Reflex loss
C4	C3–4	Trapezius, scalene	Shoulder shrugging	None
C5	C4–5	Deltoid, biceps, brachioradialis	Shoulder abduction, external rotation of arm, elbow flexion	Biceps, brachioradialis
C6	C5–6	Brachioradialis, biceps, pronator teres, extensor carpi radialis	Elbow flexion, arm pronation, finger and wrist extension	Biceps, brachioradialis
		Radial nerve injuries produce similar findings except brachioradialis function is normal		
C7	C6–7	Triceps, pronator teres, extensor digitorum	Elbow extension, finger and wrist extension	Triceps
C8	C7–T1	Flexor digitorum, flexor/ abductor pollicis, interossei	Long flexors of fingers, intrinsics of hand (finger abduction, palmar abduction of thumb)	Finger flexor
		Ulnar nerve injuries similar but also weaken thumb adductor		
T10	T9–10	—	Beevor's sign (sit-up → umbilicus pulled upward)	—
L2	L1–2	Iliopsoas	Hip flexion	Cremaster
L3	L2–3	Iliopsoas, adductors	Hip flexion, thigh adduction	Knee jerk
L4	L3–4	Quadriceps, sartorius, tibialis anterior	Knee extension, ankle dorsiflexion and inversion	Knee jerk
		Femoral nerve injury limited to knee extension; associated hip flexion and adduction weakness localizes to plexus		
L5	L4–5	Glutei, hamstrings, tibialis, extensor hallux/ digiti, peronei	Thigh adduction and internal rotation, knee flexion, plantar and dorsiflexion of ankle and toes	None
		Deep peroneal nerve weakness limited to ankle/toe extensors; posterior tibial nerve lesions weaken foot inversion		
S1	L5–S1	Gluteus maximus, hamstrings, soleus, gastrocnemius, extensor digitorum, flexor digitorum	Hip extension, knee flexion, plantar flexion of ankle and toes	Ankle jerk
S2	S1–2	Interossei	Cupping and fanning of toes	—

Reproduced with permission from the *Tarascon Internal Medicine & Critical Care Pocketbook*, 4th Edition, Tarascon Publishing.

    phenothiazines, phenytoin, procainamide, quinidine, quinine, tricyclic antidepressants, and trihexyphenidyl)
- **Management of myasthenic crisis**
  - Rapid sequence intubation with etomidate; add **low-dose** rocuronium (if necessary)
  - Plasma exchange × 5 sessions or IVIG 0.4 g/kg/d × 5 d

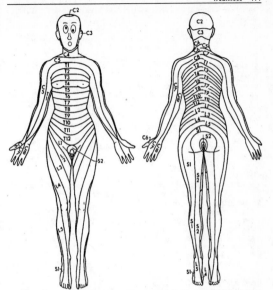

Motor level	Motor function
C1–2	neck flexion
C3	side neck flexion
C4	spontaneous breathing
C5	shoulder abduction/deltoid
C6	biceps (elbow flexion), wrist extension
C7	triceps, wrist flexion
C8	thumb extension, ulnar deviation
C8/T1	finger flexion
T1–12	intercostal and abdominal muscles

Motor level	Motor function
T7–L1	abdominal muscles
T12	cremasteric reflex
L1/L2	hip flexion, psoas
L2/3/4	hip adduction, quads
L4	foot dorsiflexion, foot inversion
L5	great toe dorsiflexion
S1	foot plantar flexion
	foot eversion
S2–4	rectal tone

Figure 12-3 Dermatomal Map
Reproduced with permission from the *Tarascon Adult Emergency Pocketbook*, 3rd Edition, Tarascon Publishing.

Table 12-8 Causes of Peripheral Neuropathies (mnemonic = MOVESTUPID)

Metabolic	B_{12}, thiamine, pyridoxine, or folate deficiencies
Other	Rare familial disorders, Amyloidosis
Vasculitis	Systemic lupus erythematosus, Sjogren, cryoglobulinemia, or polyarteritis nodosa
Endocrine	Diabetes or hypothyroidism
Syphilis or Sarcoidosis	
Tumor-related	Paraneoplastic
Uremia	Blood urea nitrogen usually >100 mg/dL
Paraproteinemia	Or porphyria or polycythemia vera
Infectious/idiopathic	Lyme disease, leprosy, mononucleosis, AIDS, or chronic inflammatory demyelinating polyneuropathy

Drugs/Toxins: alcohol, amiodarone, arsenic, β-lactams, chloroquine, carboplatin, cisplatin, colchicine, dapsone, didanosine, disulfiram, fluoroquinolones, herbicides, hydralazine, isoniazid, lead, mercury, metronidazole, niacin, nitrofurantoin, pentazocine, pesticides, phenytoin, statins, stavudine, suramin, tacrolimus, taxanes, thalidomide, vincristine, zalcitabine, and zidovudine

> Evaluate for and treat any underlying infection
> No role for anticholinesterase inhibitor therapy or steroids **during an acute crisis**
> Consider a thymectomy once the patient is stable

Multiple Sclerosis Exacerbations
- **Clinical presentation:** the presentation can vary from focal weakness, numbness, paresthesias, impaired vision, diplopia, imbalance, or impaired coordination
- **Diagnosis:** history of 2 or more neurologic deficits localized to the brain or spinal cord separated in time and space; MRI with enhancing plaques; CSF with oligoclonal bands, increased IgG index, and no pleocytosis
- **Management:** evaluate and treat any precipitating infection
  > Methylprednisolone 1 g IV daily × 3–5 d then prednisone 1 mg/kg/d × 11 d then taper

Wound Botulism
- **Clinical presentation:** diplopia, blurred vision, ptosis, dysarthria, dysphagia, dysphonia, poor gag, descending flaccid paralysis, +/– abdominal pain, nausea, vomiting, and diarrhea
- **Diagnosis:** confirmation by detecting *C. botulinum* toxin in serum and tissues
- **Treatment:** immediate wide excision and debridement of all skin wounds
  > Administer trivalent A-B-E equine antitoxin obtained from the public health department ASAP
  > Administer penicillin G 4 million units IV q4h
  > Avoid aminoglycosides, tetracyclines, and magnesium (augments neuromuscular blockade)
  > Consider early tracheostomy and gastrostomy tube placement for inability to handle oral secretions or if forced vital capacity (FVC) <15 mL/kg

References: JAMA 1998;279:859–863; Semin Neurol 2004;24:155–163; Emerg Med Clin N Am 1999;17(1):265; Am Fam Physician 2005;71:1327; South Med J 2008;101:63; Am Fam Physician 2004;70:1935; Clin Neuropharmacol 2006;29:45; and Curr Opin Neurol 2008;21: 547–562.

Section 13
Oncology

ADVERSE EFFECTS OF CHEMOTHERAPEUTIC AGENTS

- **Allergic/hypersensitivity reactions:** asparaginase, bleomycin, cetuximab, carboplatin, cisplatin, dacarbazine, daunorubicin, docetaxel, doxorubicin, etoposide, oxaliplatin, paclitaxel, procarbazine, rituximab, teniposide, and trastuzumab
- **Alopecia:** busulfan, cisplatin, cyclophosphamide, dactinomycin, daunorubicin, docetaxel, doxorubicin, etoposide, fluorouracil, idarubicin, ifosfamide, irinotecan, mitoxantrone, paclitaxel, vinblastine, vincristine, and vinorelbine
- **Cardiomyopathy:** daunorubicin, doxorubicin, epirubicin, idarubicin, mitoxantrone, sunitinib, and trastuzumab
- **Constipation:** nilutamide, thalidomide, vinblastine, vincristine, and vinorelbine
- **Diarrhea:** bicalutamide, capecitabine, cetuximab, dacarbazine, erlotinib, fluorouracil, flutamide, irinotecan, and methotrexate
- **Severe extravasation reactions:** cisplatin, daunorubicin, doxorubicin, epirubicin, etoposide, idarubicin, mechlorethamine, mitomycin C, oxaloplatin, paclitaxel, teniposide, vinblastine, vincristine, vindesine, and vinorelbine
- **Gynecomastia:** bicalutamide, estramustine, flutamide, goserelin, ketoconazole, leuprolide, nilutamide, and triptorelin
- **Hemorrhagic cystitis:** cyclophosphamide and ifosfamide
- **Hepatotoxicity:** asparaginase, bicalutamide, carmustine, cytarabine, dacarbazine, estramustine, etoposide, flutamide, gemcitabine, ifosfamide, irinotecan, ketoconazole, lomustine, mercaptopurine, methotrexate, mitomycin, nilutamide, plicamycin, streptozocin, tamoxifen, and thioguanine
- **Hypogonadism:** bleomycin, cisplatin, cyclophosphamide, epirubicin, estramustine, goserelin, ifosfamide, ketoconazole, leuprolide, triptorelin, vinblastine, vincristine, vindesine, and vinorelbine
- **Myelosuppression:** busulfan, carboplatin, carmustine, cisplatin, cyclophosphamide, cytarabine, dacarbazine, daunorubicin, doxorubicin, etoposide, bolus fluorouracil, idarubicin, ifosfamide, interferon-α, melphalan, 6-mercaptopurine, methotrexate, mitoxantrone, oxaliplatin, paclitaxel, streptozocin, taxanes, and vinblastine
- **Nephrotoxicity:** carboplatin, carmustine, cisplatin, ifosfamide, lomustine, methotrexate, mitomycin C, plicamycin, and streptozocin
- **CNS Neurotoxicity:** altretamine, asparaginase, bevacizumab, carmustine, cisplatin, cytarabine, etoposide, fluorouracil, ifosfamide, interferon-α, methotrexate, and procarbazine
- **Ototoxicity:** carboplatin, cisplatin, vinblastine, vincristine, and vinorelbine
- **Palmar-plantar dysesthesia:** capecitabine, cytarabine, fluorouracil, irinotecan, liposomal doxorubicin, sunitinib, and sorafenib
- **Peripheral/autonomic neuropathy:** altretamine, bortezomib, carboplatin, cisplatin, docetaxel, fluorouracil, ifosfamide, ixabepilone, oxaliplatin, paclitaxel, procarbazine, thalidomide, vinblastine, vincristine, and vinorelbine
- **Pulmonary toxicity:** aldesleukin, bleomycin, busulfan, carmustine, chlorambucil, cyclophosphamide, cytarabine, fludarabine, gemcitabine, melphalan, methotrexate, and procarbazine
- **Skin rashes/discoloration:** bleomycin, busulfan, cetuximab, docetaxel, doxorubicin, epirubicin, erlotinib, fluorouracil, gemcitabine, ketoconazole, and trastuzumab

- **Stomatitis/mucositis:** bleomycin, capecitabine, cytarabine, dactinomycin, daunorubicin, doxorubicin, fluorouracil, idarubicin, irinotecan, methotrexate, mitoxantrone, and oxaliplatin
- **Syndrome of inappropriate antidiuretic hormone secretion:** cisplatin, cyclophosphamide, ifosfamide, vinblastine, vincristine, and vinorelbine
- **Severe vomiting:** carmustine, carboplatin, cisplatin, cyclophosphamide, cytarabine, dacarbazine, dactinomycin, doxorubicin, dactinomycin, etoposide, ifosfamide, lomustine, mechlorethamine, high-dose methotrexate, procarbazine, and streptozocin

ONCOLOGICAL EMERGENCIES

Malignant Spinal Cord Compression
- Patients with known cancer who develop acute lower extremity neurologic deficits or fecal incontinence have cord compression until proven otherwise
  > Urgent spine MRI of cancer patients with acute back pain—rule out vertebral metastases
- Prostate, lung, and breast cancers most commonly cause cord compression
  > Less common causes: renal cell, myeloma, and non-Hodgkin lymphoma
- Thoracic (70%), lumbar (20%), cervical spine (10%), and 30% with multiple sites
- Management: dexamethasone 40 mg IV × 1 then 10 mg IV q6h; emergent MRI of entire spine; emergent neurosurgical decompression or focal radiation to spine

Brain Metastases
- Clinical presentation: headache (50%), focal weakness (40%), cognitive impairment (75%), gait disturbance (25%), seizure (15%), and behavioral changes (30%)
- Causes: lung > breast > melanoma > colon > leukemia/lymphoma > renal cell > germ cell
- Management: dexamethasone 20 mg IV × 1 then 10 mg IV q6h
- Imaging: urgent MRI of brain with and without gadolinium
- Radiation oncology and neurosurgery consultations

Superior Vena Cava Syndrome
- Clinical presentation: dyspnea (75%); cough, facial swelling and plethora; and venous distension of neck and chest wall (70%)
- Causes: lung cancer, lymphoma, and mediastinal germ cell tumor or a venous clot around a central vascular access device (10% of all cases)
- Must also rule out malignant pericardial effusion with tamponade
- Tissue diagnosis via lymph node biopsy, bronchoscopy, mediastinoscopy, or thoracotomy
- Emergent medical and radiation oncology consultations and urgent radiation therapy

Altered Mental Status in Known Cancer Patient
- Differential diagnosis: brain mets, meningitis, stroke, paraneoplastic syndrome, hypoxia, hypercalcemia, hyponatremia (usually SIADH), sepsis, hyperviscosity, or medication effect
- Treatment of hypercalcemic crisis: isotonic saline and furosemide; bisphosphonates (pamidronate 90 mg IV over 24 hr or zoledronic acid 4 mg IV over 15 min); calcitonin
  > Prednisone 40 mg/d, or its equivalent, is effective for hematologic malignancies
  > Consider gallium nitrate 200 mg/m² IV daily × 5 d for refractory hypercalcemia
- Treatment of SIADH: fluid restriction and demeclocycline 300–600 mg PO bid
  > Conivaptan 20 mg IV load then continuous drip 40 mg/d × 4 d for refractory cases

Hyperviscosity Syndrome
- Clinical presentation: mucosal bleeding, visual changes, headache, confusion, altered mental status, ataxia, vertigo, and seizures
- Causes: Waldenström macroglobulinemia, myeloma, and leukemias
- Treatment: urgent plasmapheresis or leukopheresis and hematology consultation

Tumor Lysis Syndrome (TLS)
- Clinical presentation: nausea, weakness, myalgias, dark urine, and arrhythmias
- Causes: cell lysis from chemo- or radiation therapy (usually with high-grade lymphomas; acute leukemias; CML in blast crisis; bulky, metastatic germ cell tumor of testis)
- Markedly elevated LDH correlates with risk of TLS; if LDH < 1000, TLS is unlikely
- Metabolic abnormalities: hyperuricemia, hyperkalemia, hyperphosphatemia, +/– acute kidney injury
- Standard therapy: IV hydration; allopurinol 300 mg PO bid; and keep urine pH ≥ 7
  - Rasburicase 0.2 mg/kg/d IV if uric acid >8 or creatinine >1.6 after 2 d of standard therapy
  - May need temporary hemodialysis for severe, refractory tumor lysis syndrome

Pericardial Tamponade
- Clinical presentation: dyspnea, fatigue, distant heart sounds, distended neck veins, tachycardia, hypotension, narrow pulse pressure, and pulsus paradoxus
- Causes: metastatic lung or breast CA, melanoma, leukemia, or lymphoma
- Treatment: pericardiocentesis followed by a subxiphoid pericardiotomy

Neutropenic Fever
- Neutropenia (ANC < 500) plus a fever (T $\geq$ 38°C) is infection until proven otherwise
- Evaluation: CBCD, urinalysis with micro, CXR, urine culture, blood cultures
  - Stool culture and *C. difficile* toxin only if diarrhea present
- Empiric therapy
  - Monotherapy with ceftazidime or cefepime for hemodynamically stable patients with no significant comorbidities and no clear source of fever
  - Add vancomycin if hypotensive, an indwelling catheter, severe mucositis, or a history of fluoroquinolone prophylaxis; discontinue if cultures negative at 48 hr
  - Add filgrastim 5 mcg/kg/d SQ until ANC $\geq$ 500; although benefit is unclear
  - Add antifungal therapy for persistent fevers >3 d or decompensation on antibiotics: amphotericin B, caspofungin, micafungin, anidulafungin, voriconazole, or posaconazole
  - Duration of therapy: 14 d for any bacteremia; if cultures negative, continue therapy until patient afebrile and ANC > 500 cells/μL
  - If cultures are positive, continue broad-spectrum antibiotics until ANC > 500 cells/μL, then narrow based on sensitivities of cultured organism

OTHER GENERAL RULES OF THUMB FOR CLINICAL ONCOLOGY

- Dyspnea in a cancer patient: consider pulmonary embolus, malignant pleural effusion, or postobstructive pneumonia
- Never use granulocyte colony-stimulating factors and chemotherapy concurrently

MANAGEMENT OF COMMON CHEMOTHERAPY- OR RADIATION-ASSOCIATED PROBLEMS

- Nausea and vomiting—acute
  - Mild–moderate: metoclopramide or prochlorperazine +/– lorazepam

> Severe: ondansetron, granisetron, or dolasetron +/– dexamethasone
- **Nausea and vomiting—delayed:** dexamethasone 8 mg IV bid × 48 hr **AND** metoclopromide
- **Anorexia and weight loss**
  > Trial of megestrol 80–160 mg PO qid or dronabinol 2.5–10 mg PO bid
  > Screen for depression and start antidepressants if needed
- **Bone pain**
  > Focal bone pain: external beam radiation therapy with/without opioids
  > Diffuse bone pain: bisphosphonates (if breast CA, prostate CA, or multiple myeloma); hormonal therapy; Strontium-89 with opioids; NSAIDs; or corticosteroids
- **Neuropathic pain (without neurologic deficits)**
  > Tricyclic antidepressants, gabapentin, SSRIs, opioids, and pregabalin
  > Refractory pain: consider nerve blocks; intrathecal opioids; or epidural steroids
- **Fatigue**
  > Assess for anemia, depression, malnutrition, premature menopause, side effect of chemotherapy or radiation therapy, or underlying sleep disorders
  > Regular exercise program essential; +/– methylphenidate 5 mg PO bid–tid
- **Diarrhea**
  > Rule out *Clostridium-difficile* colitis by checking stool for *C. difficile* toxin × 3
  > If *C. difficile* negative, use loperamide or diphenoxylate/atropine as needed
- **Chronic constipation oral therapy**
  > Senna 1–2 tabs daily–bid, colace 100 mg bid +/– lactulose 30 mL daily–bid
- **Alopecia**
  > Shave remaining hair from head; consider using a wig or scarves
- **Chemotherapy-induced anemia**
  > Epoetin-α or darbepoetin-α with iron to keep hemoglobin 10–11 g/dL
  > Avoid use of erythropoietic agents in cancer patients **not** receiving chemotherapy
- **Mucositis or stomatitis**
  > Compounded mixture of viscous lidocaine/diphenhydramine/sucralfate as needed
  > Gelclair: rinse mouth with 1 packet tid as needed
- **Radiation-induced thrush or odynophagia (possibly candidal esophagitis)**
  > Oral fluconazole 200 mg × 1 → 100 mg daily × 7 d (thrush) or × 3 weeks (esophagitis)
- **Dry mouth (secondary to head and neck radiation therapy)**
  > Pilocarpine 5 mg PO qid as needed
- **Radiation-induced pneumonitis**
  > Consider prednisone 30–60 mg PO daily for 2–3 weeks, then taper
- **Obstructive uropathy with urinary retention**
  > α₁-blockers: alfuzosin, doxazosin*, tamsulosin, and terazosin*
- **Radiation-induced proctitis**
  > Hydrocortisone creams, steroid enemas, or mesalamine suppositories
  > Hyperbaric oxygen therapy may be helpful for refractory cases

References: Am Fam Physician 2006;74:1873–1880; Am Fam Physician 2007;75:1207–1214; and NEJM 2000;343:1086–1094.

* generics available.

Section 14
Psychiatry

SOMATOFORM DISORDERS

Classification of Somatoform Disorders
- **Somatization disorder:** chronic disorder characterized by many recurring physical symptoms for which no organic explanation can be found; onset age <30 yr
  - History of ≥2 GI, 1 sexual, 1 pseudo-neurologic, and 4 pain symptoms involving different sites of the body
  - The symptoms are an unconscious expression of psychological distress
  - The symptoms are not intentionally produced or feigned
- **Undifferentiated somatoform disorder**
  - Duration >6 months
  - One or more unexplained physical symptoms (e.g., false pregnancy)
- **Functional somatic syndromes:** a **single** symptom for which no organic explanation can be found; not intentionally produced or feigned
  - Noncardiac chest pain, benign palpitations, irritable bowel syndrome, nonulcer dyspepsia, fibromyalgia, multiple chemical sensitivity, chronic fatigue syndrome, globus syndrome, chronic benign headache, atypical facial pain, and chronic pelvic pain
- **Hypochondriasis:** preoccupation that experienced physical sensations represent a serious disease, which persists despite medical reassurance to the contrary

Table 14-1 Differentiating Somatization Disorder and Hypochondriasis

Category	Somatization Disorder	Hypochondriasis
Gender	Women >> men	Women = men
Age of onset	Teenage years	Early adulthood
Illness beliefs	Acute sickness, disability	Serious or terminal illness
Somatic symptoms	Multiple, vague, and symptoms involve many organs	Exaggeration of normal human sensations
Preoccupations	Neglect and mistreatment by healthcare professionals	Body vulnerability and external threats to body
Illness behavior	Seeks diagnosis to legitimize sick role	Seeks reassurance about threats to health
Illness effect	Display of suffering and distress related to symptoms	Fear of serious illness and its potential consequences
Psychological symptoms	Depression	Anxiety, phobias, and obsessive-compulsive
Personality type	Dramatic and histrionic	Controlled and perfectionist
Family predilection	Somatization disorder in women Antisocial personality in men	No predilection of hypochondriasis in families

Adapted from *Lancet* 2007;369:946; *Curr Opin Psych* 2006;19:413; and *Am Fam Physician* 2007;76:1333.

- **Conversion disorder** (or "hysteria"): presents with a neurologic symptom (paralysis, amnesia, stupor, sensory loss, or pseudoseizure) that cannot be explained by an organic disorder; illness not feigned; patient may exhibit indifference or apathy about the neurologic deficit ("*la belle indifférence*")

- **Psychogenic pain disorder:** persistent pain in a single area that cannot be explained by an organic process; preoccupation is with pain and not with the underlying disease, which differentiates this disorder from hypochondriasis
- **Body dysmorphic disorder:** an unhealthy and disabling preoccupation with an imagined or minute defect in physical appearance

References: Psychother Psychosom 2006;75:270; J Psychosom Res 2004;56:455; Lancet 2007;369:946; Curr Opin Psych 2006;19:413; Emer Med J 2006;23:595; and Am Fam Physician 2007;76:1333.

MALINGERING AND FACTITIOUS DISORDERS

Malingering

- Conscious feigning, exaggeration, or self-induction of illness
- Motivation is the acquisition of some secondary gain
  - ➢ Secondary gain may mean receiving monies or disability benefits; obtaining medications of abuse; avoiding work, military duty, or incarceration; or simply accessing a warm, dry hospital bed with food
- Feigned illness may be physical or psychological in nature
  - ➢ Feigned mental illness is typically encountered in civil or criminal cases
- Patients often have a concomitant antisocial personality disorder
- Diagnosis of exclusion

Clues to the Diagnosis of Malingering

- Symptoms do not improve with treatment
- Severity of symptoms exceeds what is typical for the illness
- Weakness in the exam not seen in other activities
- Purported disability disproportionate to that seen by objective exam
- Presence of any Waddell signs: marked skin tenderness to light touch; nonanatomic tenderness to deep palpation in multiple areas; axial loading on skull causes low back pain; shoulder and pelvis rotated in same direction induces pain, difference in straight leg raising test in supine versus sitting position; sensory loss in nondermatomal distribution; overreaction to standard exam
- Evidence of self-induced illness
- Evidence of "doctor shopping," treatment in multiple municipalities, and use of multiple pharmacies
- Requests to contact family members, friends, or previous physicians are denied
- Reported history is not consistent with objective findings or laboratory data
- Vigorous opposition to psychiatric assessment and treatment
- Evidence for external incentives related to illness or incapacity
- Most common ailments to be feigned: head injury, cervical pain, repetitive strain injury, fibromyalgia, chronic fatigue syndrome, neurotoxic exposure, electrical injury, seizure disorder, and chronic abdominal or back pain

Factitious Disorders (e.g., Munchausen syndrome or Munchausen by proxy)

- Conscious production of symptoms or illness in order to assume the "sick role" and lying about the self-inflicted nature of the illness
- Requests to contact family members, friends, or previous physicians are denied
- Frequently associated with substance abuse and/or a personality disorder
- The distinguishing characteristic between malingering and factitious disorders is the motivation: malingerers are motivated by some secondary gain whereas those with factitious disorder want to assume the "sick role"
- Often elaborate stories with exaggerated lying (pseudologia fantastica)

- Patients with a factitious disorder welcome the opportunity to undergo medical or surgical procedures; conversely, malingerers aim to minimize medical testing or interventions that may uncover their deception
- Diagnosis of exclusion

References: Psych Clinics N Am *2007;30:645;* J Royal Soc Med *2007;100:81;* Psychosomatics *2006;47:23;* and Clinic Occup Environ Med *2006;5:435.*

ANTIDEPRESSANTS, ANTIPSYCHOTICS, ANXIOLYTICS

Table 14-2 Comparison of Antidepressant Medications

Name	Orthostatic hypotension	Sedation	Anticholinergic	Insomnia or agitation	GI upset, diarrhea, and nausea	Sexual dysfunction
Selective serotonin reuptake inhibitors						
citalopram	None	Some	None	Low–moderate	Moderate	Moderate
escitalopram	None	None	None	Low–moderate	Moderate	Moderate
fluoxetine	None	None	None	Moderate–high	Moderate–high	Moderate–high
fluvoxamine	None	Low	None	Low–moderate	Moderate	Moderate
paroxetine	None	Some	Low	Low–moderate	Moderate (low for Paxil CR)	Moderate–high
sertraline	None	None	None	Moderate	Moderate	Moderate
Mixed noradrenergic/serotonergic agonist antidepressants						
bupropion	None	None	None	Moderate	Low	None–low
mirtazapine	Low	Very high	Moderate	None	Low	Low
venlafaxine	None	Low	Low	Moderate	Moderate	Moderate
Tricyclic tertiary amines	High	High	High	Low	Low	Low
Tricyclic secondary amines	Moderate	Moderate	Moderate	Low	Low	Low

Continued

Table 14-2 (Continued)

Name	Other uses/miscellaneous comments	Comments
Selective serotonin reuptake inhibitors (SSRIs)		
citalopram	Panic attack and neuropathic pain/minimal drug interactions	SSRI side effects: • Headache, diarrhea, constipation, tremor, nausea, and sweating • Sexual dysfunction • Serotonin syndrome from drug interactions consists of following tetrad: ▲ Delirium ▲ Autonomic instability ▲ Neuromuscular dysfunction ▲ Fever • Discontinuation syndrome: flu-like symptoms, vertigo, emesis, and migraine HA (low risk with fluoxetine)
escitalopram	Generalized anxiety disorder/minimal drug interactions	
fluoxetine	Obsessive compulsive or premenstrual dysphoric disorder, bulimia, and panic disorder/most activating SSRI and longest drug half-life	
fluvoxamine	Obsessive compulsive disorder/long drug half-life and more nausea	
paroxetine	Obsessive compulsive, post-traumatic stress, premenstrual dysphoric and generalized anxiety disorders, panic disorder, social phobia, and neuropathic pain	
sertraline	Obsessive compulsive disorder, panic attacks, post-traumatic stress disorder, panic disorder and premenstrual dysphoric disorder	
Mixed noradrenergic/serotonergic agonist antidepressants		
bupropion	Smoking cessation	Avoid if seizures or eating disorder; can help anxiety and may cause less conversion to mania
mirtazapine	Generalized anxiety disorder, somatization disorder, panic disorder/useful adjunct for opiate withdrawal (especially because of its antiemetic effects)	Weight gain (less with higher doses), rare tremors, low mania induction, sedation
venlafaxine	Generalized anxiety disorder, bipolar disorder, and panic attacks; very effective for geriatric depression/minimal drug interactions	Nausea (less with long-acting formulation), headache and hypertension
Tricyclic antidepressant	Neuropathic pain, chronic pain, migraine prophylaxis; clomipramine and imipramine indicated for panic attacks	Severe overdose may lead to cardiac and neurotoxicity, orthostasis; use with caution in the elderly

Reference for medication side effects: Lexi-Comp.

Table 14-3 Comparison of Antipsychotic Medications

Name	EPS effects	Sedation	Anticholinergic ‡	Orthostasis	Comments/potential side effects
aripiprazole (A)	Very low	Very low	Low	Very low	Headache, nausea, vomiting, akathisia, and anxiety (activating agent)
chlorpromazine*	Moderate	High	Moderate	High	Photosensitivity, rare cytopenias, seizures
clozapine‡ (A)	None	High	High	High	Agranulocytosis, seizures, weight gain, hypersalivation, diabetes, and hyperlipidemia
fluphenazine	High	Low	Low	Low	GI upset, headache, edema, leucopenia, and akathisia
haloperidol*	High	Low	Low	Low	Akathisia, anxiety, lethargy, and hyperprolactinemia
olanzapine (A)	Low	Moderate	Low–moderate	Moderate	Akathisia, headache, rhinitis, weight gain, hyperglycemia, constipation, and dry mouth
perphenazine	Moderate	Moderate	Low–moderate	Low	Anorexia, rare cytopenias, hepatotoxicity
quetiapine (A)	Very low	Moderate	Low	Moderate	Agitation, headache, dry mouth, weight gain, diabetes, and hyperglycemia
risperidone (A)	Low–moderate†	Low	Very low	Moderate	Nausea, anxiety, tremor, weight gain, hyperglycemia, akathisia, and hyperprolactinemia (often markedly elevated)
thioridazine*	Moderate	High	High	High	Decreased libido, retrograde ejaculation, weight gain, and rarely retinitis pigmentosa
thiothixene*	High	Low	Low	Low	Agitation, photosensitivity, and hepatotoxicity
ziprasidone* (A)	Low	Moderate	Low	Low	Nausea, headache, and weakness

(A) = atypical antipsychotics, and the remainder are the "typical" antipsychotics. Clozaril effective in refractory schizophrenia. EPS = extrapyramidal side effects. QT = QT segment of electrocardiogram. *Drugs that can prolong the QT interval and may cause torsades de pointes. † Risperidone has low risk of EPS if daily dose <6 mg and moderate risk if ≥6 mg/d. ‡ Anticholinergic side effects: dry mouth, constipation, urinary retention, blurred vision, confusion, flushing, and possible worsening of narrow-angle glaucoma. Note: all antipsychotics (especially the typical neuroleptics) can cause parkinsonism and hyperprolactinemia (except for clozaril). All atypical antipsychotics can cause hyperglycemia and diabetes.
Reference for medication side effects: Lexi-Comp.

Table 14-4 Comparison of Anxiolytic Medications

Name	Equivalent dose	Therapeutic uses	PO dosage range	Comments/side effects
Benzodiazepines				
alprazolam	0.5 mg	PD, PDA, PTSD, SAD,	0.25–1† mg tid prn	Benzodiazepine side effects:
clonazepam	0.25 mg	Alcohol withdrawal	0.25–1† mg tid prn	Sedation, dizziness, anterograde amnesia, and physical
diazepam	5 mg	and akathisia	5–10† mg q6h prn	dependence. Best for short-term use.
lorazepam	1 mg		1–2† mg tid prn	Risk of benzodiazepine withdrawal syndrome (including seizures) with abrupt discontinuation.
Heterocyclic compounds (tricyclic antidepressants)				
clomipramine		PD, PDA, PTSD, OCD, SAD, and GAD	100–250 mg qhs	Drowsiness, anticholinergic side effects, tachycardia, nausea, EPS, seizures, MI or arrhythmias, weight gain. Caution in suicidal
imipramine		PD, PDA, PTSD, SAD, and GAD	100–200 mg qhs	patients.
Selective serotonin reuptake inhibitors				
fluoxetine		PD, OCD, and PMDD	20–60 mg daily	SSRI side effects: headache, diarrhea or constipation, tremor,
fluvoxamine		OCD	100–300 mg daily	nausea, vomiting, sweating, and sexual dysfunction. Fluoxetine is
paroxetine		PD, PDA, OCD, SAD, GAD, and PMDD	20–60 mg daily	most activating, paroxetine has anticholinergic effects, and fluvoxamine has the most nausea.
sertraline		PD, PDA, PTSD, OCD, SAD, GAD, and PMDD	100–200 mg daily	
Other anxiolytics				
buspirone		GAD	10–20 mg tid	Nausea, headache, dizziness, fatigue, and restlessness
propranolol		Performance anxiety and essential tremor	20–40 mg bid	Fatigue, bronchospasm, and sexual dysfunction
venlafaxine		GAD, SAD, and PMDD	75–225 mg XR daily	Hypertension, agitation, tremor, nausea, headache, somnolence, dizziness, dry mouth, and constipation

PD = panic disorder; PDA = panic disorder with agoraphobia; PTSD = post-traumatic stress disorder; SAD = social anxiety disorder; GAD = generalized anxiety disorder; PMDD = premenstrual dysphoric disorder; OCD = obsessive compulsive disorder; EPS = extrapyramidal side effects. Anticholinergic side effects: dry mouth, blurry vision, constipation, urinary retention, confusion, and flushing. * Indicates long half-life benzodiazepines. † ↓ dose by 50% in elderly.
Reference for medication side effects: Lexi-Comp.

Section 15
Pulmonary Medicine

MANAGEMENT OF ASTHMA EXACERBATIONS

Table 15-1 Risk Factors for Death in Asthmatics

Sudden severe attacks	Prior intubation/ICU stay	≥2 ER/hospitalizations/yr
Hospital/ER in last month	Recent systemic steroids	>2 albuterol canisters/mo
Heart/psychiatric disorder	Illicit drug use	Low socioeconomic class

Adapted from *Curr Opin Pulm Med* 2008;14:13.

Initial assessment of severity in acute asthma exacerbations in adults			
Symptoms	Mild	Moderate	Severe
Speaking in . . .	sentences	phrases	words
Heart rate (bpm)	<100	100–120	>120
PEF/FEV$_1$ (% predicted)	>75%	40–75%	<40% (especially <25%)
Room air pulse oximetry	>95%	91–95%	≤90%
Mental status	Alert	Drowsy	Lethargic/obtunded
PaCO$_2$ (mmHg)	<40	40–50	>50

Inpatient treatment of moderate–severe asthma exacerbations
- Oxygen to keep SaO$_2$ > 90%
- Albuterol 2.5 mg Neb q1h until stable; then q2h/q1h prn × 24 hr; then q4h/q2h prn
  ➤ Consider 2.5 mg Neb q 20 min × 3 or 10 mg continuous over 1 hr for severe asthma
  ➤ Albuterol and levalbuterol are equally efficacious
- Ipratropium 0.5 mg Neb q 20 min × 3 for severe asthma; then q4h/q2h prn; then q6h
- Methylprednisolone 60 mg IV q6h until bronchospasm controlled; then prednisone 1 mg/kg PO daily to complete 10–14 d of therapy then taper
- Consider magnesium 2 g IV over 20 min for severe asthma exacerbations
- Empiric antibiotics for pneumonia or bronchitis **only** if purulent sputum production

Good response after 1–2 hr
- Continue current therapy on wards
- Serial PEF and oximetry monitoring
- Smoking cessation counseling, if applicable, and patient education

Partial/poor response after 1–2 hr
- Consider noninvasive positive pressure ventilation in ICU
- Continue q1h nebulizer treatments

Reassess after 1–2 hr
- ABG
- Serial PEF and oximetry monitoring
- Consider IV aminophylline only for severe, refractory asthma (high risk of toxicity)
- Consider intubation for: persistent PaCO$_2$ > 50 with respiratory acidosis; worsening mental status; hemodynamic instability; or progressive deterioration despite maximal medical therapy
  ➤ Propofol and ketamine will bronchodilate
  ➤ Maximize expiratory time
  ➤ Keep Pplateau ≤ 30 cmH$_2$O

Figure 15-1 Management of Acute Asthma Exacerbations
PEF = peak expiratory flow rate; FEV$_1$ = forced expiratory volume at 1 sec; PaCO$_2$ = partial pressure of carbon dioxide.
Adapted from *Allergy* 2008;63:997; *Curr Opin Pulm Med* 2008;14:13; and *Clin Chest Med* 2006;27:99.

CHRONIC OBSTRUCTIVE PULMONARY DISEASE (COPD)

Table 15-2 Management of Stable COPD by Stage

Stage*	Spirometry	Therapy
All	No Smoking! Influenza and pneumococcal vaccines and exercise	
0 (at risk)	Normal	
I (mild)	$FEV_1/FVC < 70\%$ $FEV_1 \geq 80\%$ predicted	Short-acting or long-acting β_2-agonist or anticholinergic (AC) agent† prn
II (moderate)	$FEV_1/FVC < 70\%$ $50\% \leq FEV_1 < 80\%$	Scheduled long-acting β_2-agonist or AC agent† and pulmonary rehabilitation‡
III (severe)	$FEV_1/FVC < 70\%$ $30\% \leq FEV_1 < 50\%$	Add inhaled steroids to scheduled long-acting bronchodilators (especially if ≥1 exacerbations per year)
IV (very severe)	$FEV_1 < 30\%$ or $<50\%$ + chronic resp failure	As for stage III; oxygen§ (improves survival!); consider bullectomy/transplant‖

resp = respiratory.
* FEV_1 used to stratify severity. BODE index (body mass index, airway obstruction, dyspnea, exercise capacity on 6 min walk) better to assess risk of death; see http://content.nejm.org/cgi/reprint/350/10/1005.pdf.
† Bronchodilators (anticholinergics > β_2-agonists >> methylxanthines): use combination therapy if monotherapy inadequate; long-acting anticholinergic (tiotropium) and β_2-agonist (e.g., salmeterol or formoterol) are preferred over short-acting anticholinergic (ipratropium) or β_2-agonist (e.g., albuterol).
‡ Aerobic exercise, good nutrition, and education.
§ Indications for supplemental oxygen: $PaO_2 \leq 55$ mmHg/O_2 stat ≤88% ($PaO_2 \leq 60$ mmHg if pulmonary hypertension, polycythemia, or cor pulmonale).
‖ Bullectomy or lung-volume reduction surgery best for upper lobe emphysema and low exercise capacity.
Note: Lung transplantation indicated for idiopathic emphysema or α-1 antitrypsin deficiency.
Adapted from the GOLD initiative 2007 executive summary available at www.goldcopd.com.

Acute COPD Exacerbations (increase in dyspnea, cough, sputum volume, or purulence)
- Assess with CXR, sputum culture, oximetry, or arterial blood gas
- Admit for moderate–severe exacerbations: respiratory acidosis, need for ventilation, PEF < 100 L/min, $FEV_1 < 1$ L or < 40% predicted, or serious comorbidities
- **Medical management of acute COPD exacerbations**
  ➤ Albuterol 2.5 mg and ipratropium 0.5 mg nebulized q2–4 hr
  ➤ Antibiotics × 5–10 d for severe exacerbations or presence of purulent sputum
    ○ Uncomplicated exacerbation if age ≤65 yr, $FEV_1 \geq 50\%$ and <4 exacerbations/yr—use new macrolide, doxycycline, or 2nd- or 3rd-generation cephalosporin
    ○ Complicated exacerbation if age >65 yr, $FEV_1 < 50\%$, >4 exacerbations/yr, or use of antibiotics in the last 3 months—use amoxicillin–clavulanate or a respiratory quinolone
    ○ Risk for pseudomonas if recurrent antibiotic use, recurrent steroid courses, or if bronchiectasis is present; use an antipseudomonal quinolone
  ➤ Systemic steroids with methylprednisolone 30–40 mg/d or (prednisone 40–60 mg PO daily) × 7–10 d if $FEV_1 < 50\%$ predicted, **or** if $PaCO_2 > 45$ and pH < 7.35 +/– steroid taper

> Oxygen if hypoxia to maintain SaO_2 88–90% or $PaO_2 \geq 55$ mmHg
> Noninvasive positive-pressure ventilation if acute respiratory acidosis (pH ≤ 7.35, $PaCO_2 \geq 45$ mmHg) and no contraindications to its use
- Indications for ICU admission: $PaCO_2 > 60$ mmHg and pH < 7.25; depressed level of consciousness; unstable medical comorbidities; hemodynamic or rhythm instability; and need for invasive mechanical ventilation
- Indications for mechanical ventilation: severe respiratory acidosis refractory to noninvasive ventilation; respiratory arrest; hemodynamic instability; or obtundation

References: GOLD initiative at www.goldcopd.com; Am J Med 2006;119:S46; Am J Med 2007;120:S4; Ann Fam Med 2007;4:253; Lancet 2004;364:883; and Chest 2008;133:756.

EVALUATION OF PLEURAL EFFUSION

Table 15-3 Classification of Pleural Effusions

Test	Transudate	Exudate[†]
Serum-PF albumin gradient*	>1.2 g/dL	$\leq$1.2 g/dL
PF protein/serum protein	$\leq$0.5	>0.5
PF LDH (international units)	<2/3 upper limit of labs normal range (or $\leq$ 130)	>2/3 upper limit of labs normal range (or >130)
PF LDH/serum LDH	$\leq$0.6	>0.6

PF = pleural fluid; LDH = lactate dehydrogenase.
* Useful to diagnose transudative effusions after patient has received diuretics.
† **Only 1 test needs to be abnormal to classify effusion as an exudate.**
Note: PF glucose <60 suggests cancer, tuberculosis, empyema, or effusion from lupus or rheumatoid lung.
Adapted from *N Engl J Med* 2002;346:1971–1977.

Table 15-4 Causes of Transudative Effusions

• Constrictive pericarditis	• Hepatic hydrothorax	• Nephrotic syndrome	• Severe hypoalbuminemia*
• Urinothorax	• Heart Failure*	• Peritoneal dialysis	• Superior vena cava syndrome

* Most common causes of transudative pleural effusions.
Adapted from *N Engl J Med* 2002;346:1971–1977.

Contraindications to Diagnostic Thoracentesis
- International normalized ratio >2.0 or partial thromboplastin time greater than twice normal
  > Can perform thoracentesis if coagulopathy corrected prior to procedure
- Platelets <50,000 cells/mL
- Caution if blood urea nitrogen >80 mg/dL
- Small volume of pleural fluid: <1 cm pleural fluid on a decubitus CXR
  > Thoracentesis can be done **if free-flowing fluid > 1 cm** on a decubitus CXR

References: Am Fam Physician 2006;73:1211–1220 and NEJM 2002;346:1971–1977.

Table 15-5 Evaluation of Exudative Effusions

Diagnosis	PF appearance	Diagnostic pleural fluid testing
Empyema	Purulent	PF pH < 7.2*, ↑ WBC†, glucose < 40 mg/dL, and culture
Malignant	+/− Bloody	Positive pleural fluid cytology
Chylothorax	Milky	Triglycerides >110 mg/dL
Pancreatitis	—	High amylase
Uremia	—	BUN (usually >100 mg/dL)
Sarcoidosis	—	High angiotensin-converting enzyme level
Lupus pleuritis	—	Positive pleural fluid antinuclear antibody (ANA)
Rheumatoid lung	Yellow-green	Characteristic cytology, glucose <30 mg/dL
Ovarian hyperstimulation syndrome	—	Fertility medication use
Meig syndrome	—	Ascites and ovarian fibroma present
Amebic abscess	Anchovy paste	Elevated amebic titers and liver abscess present
Pulmonary embolus	Bloody	Positive CT pulmonary angiogram or V/Q scan
Tuberculosis	Bloody	Positive acid fast bacilli (AFB) on pleural biopsy and <5% mesothelial cells in pleural fluid AFB RNA by PCR (40–80% sensitive); adenosine deaminase >40 units/L (90% sensitive)

PF = pleural fluid; V/Q = ventilation/perfusion; WBC = white blood cells.
* Fluid for pleural fluid pH should be collected in a lithium heparin tube and kept on ice.
† ↑ WBC = pleural fluid white blood count >25,000 cell/μL (collect in a purple top tube).
• Pleural fluid lymphocytosis >50%: 90–96% secondary to either malignancy or tuberculosis
• Pleural fluid pH < 7.2: empyema, malignancy, tuberculosis, ruptured esophagus, urinothorax, lupus pleuritis, or rheumatoid lung
• Bloody pleural effusion: trauma, malignancy, pulmonary embolus, tuberculosis, or traumatic tap
• Any effusion that develops during pneumonia treatment should be aspirated and analyzed.
Adapted from *Am Fam Physician* 2006;73:1211.

PNEUMOTHORAX

Primary Spontaneous Pneumothorax (PSP)
• Risk factors: thin, tall men (10–30 yr); smoking; mitral valve prolapse; and Marfan syndrome

Secondary Spontaneous Pneumothorax (SSP)
• Underlying lung disease (COPD, cystic fibrosis, asthma, connective-tissue disease, DILD)
• Lung infections (necrotizing bacterial or *Pneumocystis jiroveci* pneumonia or tuberculosis)
• Catamenial pneumothorax (thoracic endometriosis)
• Cancer (sarcoma or lung cancer)

Treatment of Pneumothorax
• Pneumothorax evacuation kit connected to a Heimlich valve or a thoracic vent is adequate for any iatrogenic pneumothorax, PSP, or SSP > 15% in size that is hemodynamically stable
• Pneumothoraces (<15%) in hemodynamically stable patients can be treated with 100% oxygen and observation.

- Chest tube is necessary for any hydropneumothorax, hemopneumothorax, tension pneumothorax, or if the patient is receiving positive pressure ventilation
- Consider surgery for bullae resection or pleurodesis if recurrent spontaneous pneumothoraces

Reference: NEJM 2000;342:868–874.

INTERSTITIAL LUNG DISEASE

- **History:** occupational/environmental exposures, travel, meds, medical comorbidities
- **Diagnostic studies**
  - ➤ CXR and arterial blood gas
  - ➤ High-resolution chest CT: reticulonodular infiltrates, interstitial infiltrates, "ground glass" opacities, or honeycombing
  - ➤ Pulmonary function testing reveals a pattern of restrictive lung disease with a decline in lung volumes and diffusion capacity
  - ➤ Labs: CBCD, chem panel, angiotensin-converting enzyme, ANA, RF, antineutrophil cytoplasmic antibody, antiglomerular basement membrane antibody, anti-ScL-70, HIV, ESR, CK, HLA-B27, aldolase levels, and coccidioidomycosis titers
  - ➤ Induced sputa or bronchoalveolar lavage for cytology and AFB or fungi
  - ➤ Open lung biopsy

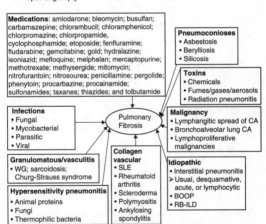

Figure 15-2 Causes of Diffuse Interstitial Lung Disease
SLE = systemic lupus erythematosus; WG = Wegener granulomatosis; BOOP = bronchiolitis obliterans with organizing pneumonia; RB-ILD = respiratory bronchiolitis-interstitial lung disease.
Adapted from *South Med J* 2007;100:579.

Treatment of Diffuse Interstitial Lung Disease (DILD)

- Targeted therapy of any underlying disease that has been identified
- Avoidance of offending medication(s) or occupational exposures if relevant
- Supplemental O_2 to keep $PaO_2 > 55$ mmHg; pneumococcal and influenza vaccines
- Idiopathic interstitial pneumonitis: prednisone 0.5–1 mg/kg/d often with cyclophosphamide 2 mg/kg PO daily **or** azathioprine 2 mg/kg PO daily
- Refer appropriate patients for lung transplantation

References: South Med J 2007;100:579; Chest 2006;129:180S; Curr Opin Pulm Med 2008;14:427; and Thorax 2008;63:v1–v58.

PULMONARY HYPERTENSION

Definition

- Mean pulmonary artery pressure >25 mmHg (rest) or >30 mmHg (exercise)
- **Pulmonary arterial hypertension (PAH):** above and normal pulmonary capillary wedge pressure or left ventricular end-diastolic pressure or normal LVEDP

Table 15-6 Classification of Pulmonary Hypertension (PHTN)

Subtypes of PHTN	Causes
Pulmonary arterial hypertension (PAH)	• Idiopathic
	• Familial
	• Associated with a connective tissue disease
	• Associated with HIV infection
	• Portopulmonary hypertension
	• Drug-induced or toxin-induced
	• Pulmonary veno-occlusive disease
	• Pulmonary capillary hemangiomatosis
PHTN with left heart disease	• Chronic CHF; Moderate–severe MS or MR
Secondary to chronic hypoxia	• COPD; DILD; OSA; obesity-hypoventilation syndrome; neuromuscular disorders; intracardiac R → L shunts
Recurrent pulmonary emboli	• Recurrent PE or tumor emboli
Miscellaneous	• Sarcoidosis; Langerhans cell histiocytosis; schistosomiasis; and lymphangiomatosis

Adapted from J Am Coll Cardiol 2004;43:5S.

Evaluation of Pulmonary Hypertension

- ECG: right axis deviation; right atrial abnormality; and right ventricular hypertrophy
- CXR: enlarged right atrium and ventricle; dilated pulmonary arteries; and "pruning" of the peripheral pulmonary vasculature
- Pulmonary function test: screen for underlying obstructive or restrictive lung disease
- Nocturnal polysomnogram: evaluate for obstructive or central sleep apnea
- Arterial blood gas: screen for resting hypoxia or hypercarbia
- V/Q scan superior to CT pulmonary angiogram to screen for recurrent PE
- Echocardiogram: evaluate left ventricular systolic and diastolic function, valve abnormalities, chamber sizes, and noninvasive estimate of pulmonary pressures
- Right heart catheterization: confirms diagnosis of pulmonary arterial hypertension
- Labs: CBCD, chem panel, ANA, RF, anti-Scl-70, anticentromere, HIV, and ESR
- Six-minute walk test to determine functional capacity

Treatment

- Supplemental oxygen to keep $SaO_2 \geq 90\%$
- Interventions: influenza and pneumococcal vaccinations; smoking cessation; chronic anticoagulation; and **avoid** decongestants, pregnancy, NSAIDs, and air travel
- Consider cautious diuresis and/or digoxin therapy for right ventricular dysfunction
- Pulmonary vasoreactivity as determined by inhaled nitric oxide testing during right heart catheterization can benefit from nifedipine ER, amlodipine, or diltiazem therapy
- Initial medication therapy for functional classes 2–3 and good hemodynamic profile
  - ➤ Endothelin receptor antagonists: bosentan or ambrisentan
  - ➤ Phosphodiesterase-5 inhibitors: sildenafil
- Initial medication therapy for functional classes 3–4 with poor hemodynamic profile
  - ➤ Prostanoid therapy: epoprostenol IV or inhaled iloprost or treprostinil SQ or IV

References: Am J Med Sci *2008;335:40;* Circulation *2008;118:2190;* Crit Care Med *2007;35:2037;* and Expert Opin Pharmacother *2008;9:65.*

HEMOPTYSIS

Table 15-7 Causes of Hemoptysis

Category	Causes
Infectious	Bronchitis; pneumonia (viral, bacterial, fungal); bronchiectasis; aspergillosis; tuberculosis
Malignancy	Primary lung cancer or lung metastases
Cardiovascular	PE; pulmonary artery rupture; CHF; mitral stenosis
Vasculitis	Wegener granulomatosis or Goodpasture syndrome
Miscellaneous	Chest trauma; foreign body; anticoagulation; epistaxis; bronchovascular fistula; pulmonary arterio-venous malformation; or Dieulafoy disease

Adapted from Arch Intern Med *1991;151:2449* and Chest *1997;112:440.*

Evaluation of Hemoptysis

- Labs: CBC, chemistry panel, PT, PTT, urinalysis, and oximetry
- CXR and CT scan of the chest (tracheal or proximal bronchial lesions missed by CXR)
- Tests to consider: sputum culture, PPD, sputum for AFB, coccidioidomycosis titer, and antineutrophil cytoplasmic and antiglomerular basement membrane antibodies
- Fiberoptic bronchoscopy indicated for unexplained hemoptysis

Management of Massive Hemoptysis

- Intubation (preferably selective intubation of normal lung) and mechanical ventilation with the affected lung kept dependent in the lateral decubitus position
- Transfuse platelets or fresh frozen plasma for thrombocytopenia or a coagulopathy
- Pulmonary angiogram and selective embolization of the bronchial artery
- Lobectomy or pneumonectomy in refractory cases

References: Chest *2008;133:212;* Curr Opin Pulm Med *2008;14:195;* and Clin Chest Med *1994;15:147.*

Section 16
Renal Medicine

ACUTE KIDNEY INJURY

Definition of Acute Kidney Injury (AKI)
• AKI should be abrupt (within 1–7 d) and sustained (>24 hr)

Table 16-1 RIFLE Classification* of Acute Kidney Injury

Class	GFR criteria	Urine output (UO) criteria
Risk	↑ serum creatinine† × 1.5	UO < 0.5 mL/kg/hr × 6 hr
Injury	↑ serum creatinine† × 2	UO < 0.5 mL/kg/hr × 12 hr
Failure (acute renal failure)	↑ serum creatinine† × 3 or ↑ >0.5 mg/dL above 4 mg/dL	UO < 0.5 mL/kg/hr × 24 hr‡
Loss	Persistent acute renal failure for more than 4 weeks	
End-stage kidney disease	Persistent renal loss for more than 3 months	

* RIFLE class is determined based on the worst of **either** GFR criteria or urine output criteria.
† Represents the **baseline** serum creatinine; GFR = glomerular filtration rate.
‡ Or anuria >12 hr.
Adapted from *Crit Care* 2006;10:73.

Causes of Acute Kidney Injury
• Causes of prerenal azotemia (55–60% of cases)
  ➢ Hypovolemia
  ➢ Distributive shock (sepsis, anaphylaxis, or neurogenic)
  ➢ Decreased effective circulating volume (chronic CHF, sepsis, nephrotic syndrome, decompensated cirrhosis, or "third spacing" of fluids)
  ➢ Decreased cardiac output (cardiogenic shock or pericardial tamponade)
  ➢ Chronic hypercalcemia causing renal vasoconstriction
  ➢ Meds: ACEIs, ARBs, NSAIDs, COX-2 inhibitors, cyclosporine, amphotericin B, radiocontrast dyes, hydralazine, and minoxidil
• Causes of postrenal or obstructive nephropathy (5–10% of cases)
  ➢ Bilateral ureteral obstruction
  ➢ Bladder outlet obstruction (benign prostatic hyperplasia; bladder stone; cancer of the cervix, bladder, or prostate; or a urethral stricture)
  ➢ Neurogenic bladder
  ➢ Crystal-forming meds: acetazolamide, acyclovir, indinavir, methotrexate, sulfadiazine, topiramate, and triamterene
• **Intrinsic AKI:** acute glomerulonephritis, tubular necrosis, or interstitial nephritis
• Causes of acute glomerulonephritis (AGN) (2–3% of cases)
  ➢ Systemic illnesses: systemic lupus erythematosus, Wegener granulomatosis, Goodpasture disease, and polyarteritis nodosa
  ➢ Henoch-Schönlein purpura or immunoglobulin A (IgA) nephropathy
  ➢ Infectious: hepatitis B and C viruses, endocarditis, HIV, post-streptococcal
  ➢ Malignancy
  ➢ Mixed cryoglobulinemia (often hepatitis C virus-related)
  ➢ Meds: allopurinol, cytokine rx, gold, hydralazine, pamidronate, penicillamine
• Causes of acute tubular necrosis (ATN) (35% of cases)
  ➢ Ischemia from renal hypoperfusion

> Meds/toxins: aminoglycosides, amphotericin B, arsenic, carboplatin, cisplatin, chromium, contrast dyes, cyclosporine, foscarnet, ifosfamide, methotrexate, methoxyflurane, oxaliplatin, pentamidine, plicamycin, rifampin, tetracyclines, and trimetrexate
> Pigment-related: severe hemolysis or rhabdomyolysis
> Cast nephropathy from multiple myeloma
- **Acute interstitial nephritis (AIN) (2–3% of cases)**
  > Meds (90% of AIN): acyclovir, adefovir, allopurinol, azathioprine, carbamazepine, cephalosporins, cidofovir, cimetidine, cyclosporine, erythromycin, ethambutol, fluoroquinolones, furosemide, lithium, NSAIDs, omeprazole, penicillins, phenobarbital, phenytoin, ranitidine, rifampin, sulfonamides, tacrolimus, tetracyclines, thiazides, trimethoprim, vancomycin, and some Chinese herbs (such as aristolochic acid)
  > Miscellaneous causes: infection, lymphomatous or leukemic infiltration
- **Other nephrotoxic agents:** cytarabine and melphalan (via tumor lysis syndrome), gemcitabine and mitomycin (hemolytic uremic syndrome), interleukin-2 (vascular leak syndrome), gallium nitrate, IV immune globulin, nitrosoureas, and streptozocin (unclear etiologies for acute renal failure)
- **Causes of pseudo-renal failure** (benign elevation of serum creatinine)
  > Cimetidine, glucocorticoids, and trimethoprim

Clinical Presentation of Acute Kidney Injury
- Asymptomatic, fatigue, lethargy, and generalized weakness
- Congestive heart failure or anasarca
- Uremia: somnolence, pericarditis, asterixis, nausea, anorexia, or pruritus

Table 16-2 Urinary Studies in Acute Kidney Injury

Subtype	Urinary sediment	UNa (mmol/L)	Protein (mg/dL)	FENa (%)	FEurea* (%)
Prerenal	Bland	<20	0	<1	<35
Postrenal	Bland	Usually >20	0	>1	>35
AGN	RBC casts	<20	≥ 100	<1	<35
ATN	Gran. casts	>20	30–100	>1†	>35
AIN	WBC casts	>20	30–100	>1	>35

U = urine; crt = creatinine; BUN = blood urea nitrogen; Na = sodium; RBC = red blood cells; WBC = white blood cells; Gran. = granular.
FENa = fractional excretion of sodium = (UNa × serum crt)/(Ucrt × serum Na) × 100
FEurea = fractional excretion of urea = (Uurea × serum crt)/(Ucrt × BUN) × 100
* More useful measure when patient receiving diuretics.
† Contrast nephropathy, sepsis, pigment-induced nephropathy, and AKI with underlying cirrhosis all can cause ATN with a FENa < 1.
Adapted from *Am Fam Physician* 2005;72:1739 and *Am Fam Physician* 2003;67:2527.

Workup of Acute Kidney Injury
- Careful effort to find any prior serum creatinine values (if possible)
- Thorough history and physical and careful investigation of medication history
- Calculate FENa or FEurea using equations above and check urinary sediment
- Place a Foley catheter and measure the postvoid residual after urine studies done
- Renal ultrasound (for size and to check for hydronephrosis/hydroureter)
- Labs to consider depending on classification of AKI and likely causes: urine eosinophils (present in 30% of AIN), complete blood count, electrolytes, renal panel,

calcium, phosphate, hepatitis B and C virus serologies, HIV test, antistreptolysin O titer, antiglomerular basement membrane antibody, antineutrophil cytoplasmic antibody, antinuclear antibody, complement studies, serum cryoglobulins, blood cultures, serum, and urine protein electrophoreses
- When to perform a renal biopsy
  - ➤ There is no unanimous consensus about this issue
  - ➤ Reasonable approach is to biopsy patients with an active urinary sediment or who have an unexplained intrarenal process (AGN, ATN, or AIN)

Prevention of Contrast-Induced Nephropathy
- Maintain adequate hydration; stop potentially nephrotoxic medications for at least 24–48 hr (e.g., ACEIs, ARBs, diuretics, and NSAIDs)
- N-acetylcysteine 600 mg PO bid × 4 doses starting a day before the procedure
- D_5W with 3 amps $NaHCO_3$ at 3 mL/kg/hr for 1 hr before the contrast and 1 mL/kg/hr for 6 hr after the contrast procedure (significant sodium load)

Indication for Acute Dialysis (mnemonic AEIOU)
A—Acidosis: persistent arterial pH < 7.2 refractory to medical therapy
E—Electrolytes: severe hyperkalemia refractory to medical therapy
I—Intoxications or overdoses
O—fluid Overload
U—Uremia

References: J Am Soc Neph 1999;10(8):1833; J Am Soc Neph 1998;9:506, 710; Crit Care 2006;10:73; Am Fam Physician 2000;61:2077; Am Fam Physician 2005;72:1739; and Am Fam Physician 2003;67:2527.

CHRONIC KIDNEY DISEASE (CKD)

KDIGO (Kidney Disease: Improving Global Outcomes) Definition of CKD
- Structural or functional kidney abnormalities or kidney transplantation for ≥3 months
  - ➤ Hematuria, proteinuria, or abnormal kidneys by imaging or laboratory studies **OR**
  - ➤ Glomerular filtration rate (GFR) < 60 mL/min/1.73 m^2 for ≥3 mo

Table 16-3 National Kidney Foundation Stages of Chronic Kidney Disease

Stage	Description	GFR* (mL/min/1.73 m^2)	Action
1	Kidney damage (NL GFR)	≥90	Treat comorbid conditions, slow progression, and CVD risk reduction
2	Mild ↓ GFR	60–89	Estimate/slow disease progression
3	Moderate ↓ GFR	30–59	Treat disease complications Referral to nephrologist[†]
4	Severe ↓ GFR	15–29	Prepare for dialysis/transplantation
5	Renal failure	<15	Dialyze if uremic or GFR < 10

CVD = cardiovascular disease; GFR = glomerular filtration rate.
* GFR calculated with the MDRD equation available at www.kidney.org/professionals/kdoqi/gfr_calculator.cfm.
† Consider nephrology referral when patients reach advanced stage 2 CKD.
Adapted from the KDOQI guidelines available at www.kdoqi.org.

Table 16-4 Select Etiologies of CKD*

• Diabetes mellitus	• Hypertension	• Polycystic kidney disease
• Glomerulonephritis	• Alport syndrome	• Medullary sponge kidney
• Reflux nephropathy	• Myeloma kidney	• Analgesic nephropathy
• Sarcoidosis	• Amyloidosis	• Chronic obstructive uropathy
• Lupus nephritis	• IgA nephropathy	• Hypercalcemic nephropathy

* DM and hypertension account for 66% of all cases.
Adapted from *NEJM* 2006;355:2088–2098 and *Ann Intern Med* 2006;145:247–254.

Screening for CKD in Adults
- Risk factors for CKD: age > 60 yr; family history of CKD; history of low birth weight; HIV, Tb, HBV, or HCV infection; diabetes; HTN; cardiovascular disease; autoimmune disease; recurrent UTIs; nephrolithiasis; certain cancers; exposure to nephrotoxic drugs; or obstructive uropathy
- All patients with risk factors for CKD should be screened annually
- Screen with urine albumin-to-creatinine ratio and estimation of GFR
  ➤ Urine albumin-to-creatinine ratio 30–300 mg/g = microalbuminuria
  ➤ Urine albumin-to-creatinine ratio > 300 mg/g = macroalbuminuria
- MDRD (Modification of Diet in Renal Disease) equation for estimating GFR to determine the stage of CKD; not validated for drug dosing in renal insufficiency
  ➤ Available at www.kidney.org/professionals/kdoqi/gfr_calculator.cfm
  ➤ Cockcroft-Gault equation is used to determine CrCl for drug dosing in CKD
- Urinalysis and microscopy to assess for hematuria, pyuria, and casts
- Renal ultrasound if obstructive uropathy, severe HTN, recurrent UTIs, or active urinary sediment

Monitoring Patients with CKD
- Follow urine protein-to-creatinine (mg/g) ratio once overt proteinuria develops
  ➤ First morning urine collection is preferred
- Monitor GFR, proteinuria, Hgb, iPTH, calcium, bicarbonate, potassium, and phosphorus
  ➤ Stages 3 CKD monitor q 6 mo; stage 4–5 CKD monitor at least every 3 mo

Screening for Diabetic Kidney Disease
- Patients with diabetes should be screened annually for diabetic nephropathy
- Screening for CKD as above 5 years after diagnosis of DM 1 and at the time DM 2 is diagnosed
- Consider other causes of CKD if: absence of DM retinopathy; rapidly decreasing GFR; refractory HTN; active urinary sediment; or signs of another systemic disease

Management of Diabetes with CKD Stages 1–4
- Target HgbA1c < 7%
- ACEI/ARB for HTN or albuminuria; BP goal <130/80 mmHg (<125/75 if proteinuria)
- Indications for treadmill or myocardial perfusion test: chest pain, possible anginal equivalent, >35 yr and plans to begin vigorous exercise, carotid artery stenosis, or peripheral vascular disease

Management of Anemia of CKD
- Epoetin-α 50–100 U/kg IV 3×/week with hemodialysis
  ➤ Target hemoglobin 11–12 g/dL; avoid hemoglobin levels >13 g/dL
- PO/IV iron to maintain transferrin saturation >20%
  ➤ Ferritin levels may be elevated due to inflammation/infection in hospitalized pts

Surgical Referrals

- Refer patient to surgeon for dialysis access when CrCl < 25 mL/min
  - Protect arm most suitable for access from venipunctures, IVs, or BP checks
- Refer for transplant evaluation once CrCl ≤ 20 mL/min even if *not* on dialysis

Metabolic Acidosis

- Maintain serum bicarbonate ≥22 mmol/L with sodium bicarbonate 0.5–1 mEq/kg/d
- May use diuretics to control hypertension, fluid retention, and hyperkalemia (which itself can cause decreased ammoniagenesis and metabolic acidosis)

Nutrition

- 2 g sodium, low potassium, and low phosphate for all patients with CKD
- 1.2 g/kg/d protein with chronic hemodialysis; 1.2–1.3 g/kg/d for peritoneal dialysis; 0.8 g/kg/d protein + urinary losses if pt has nephrotic syndrome predialysis
- Periodic assessment of predialysis albumin and weekly weight checks

Vitamins

- Initiate multivitamin 1 tablet PO daily and folic acid 1 mg PO daily

Management of Secondary Hyperparathyroidism in CKD

- Goal phosphorus 2.7–4.6 mg/dL (stage 3–4); keep 3.5–5.5 mg/dL if chronic dialysis
- Maintain serum calcium–phosphorus product <55
- Goal iPTH: stage 3 (35–70 pg/mL); stage 4 (70–110 pg/mL); stage 5 (150–300 pg/mL)
- Annual dual-energy x-ray absorptiometry in patients to rule out osteoporosis
- **Calcium phosphate binders (use if patient is hypocalcemic; avoid if calcium > 10.2 mg/dL)**
  - Calcium acetate (Phoslo) 1–3 tabs PO tid with meals; calcium carbonate is alternative (watch for premature development of vascular calcifications)
- **Vitamin D analogs** (start if ↑ iPTH + 25-hydroxyvitamin D [25-(OH)D] ≤ 30 ng/mL)
  - Calcitriol (Rocaltrol) 0.25–2 mcg PO daily **or** paricalcitol (Zemplar) 1–4 mcg PO every other day **or** doxercalciferol (Hectorol) 2–6 mcg IV/PO 3×/wk
  - Titrate dose to appropriate iPTH levels based on stage of CKD
  - Use with caution if serum calcium >9.5 mg/dL and phosphate >4.6 mg/dL

Options for refractory secondary hyperparathyroidism on dialysis (iPTH > 300 pg/mL); may use with or without vitamin D

- Cinacalcet 30–180 mg PO daily; use if calcium normal/high; also for calciphylaxis
  - Start 30 mg PO daily; titrate until iPTH 150–300 pg/mL; calcium >=9.5 mg/dL; and phosphorus <5.5 mg/dL
- Sevelamer hydrochloride 800–3200 mg PO tid with meals (option for hypercalcemia)
- Sevelamer bicarbonate 800–1600 mg PO tid with meals (option for hypercalcemia)
- Lanthanum 250–1250 mg PO tid with meals (**alternative if marked hyperphosphatemia**)
- Parathyroidectomy for severe, refractory hyperparathyroidism (iPTH > 800 pg/mL)
- Ergocalciferol 50,000 IU PO q wk–month for vitamin D deficiency (25-[OH]D < 30 ng/mL)

Lifestyle Changes

- Cessation of smoking
- Target LDL-cholesterol < 100 mg/dL; statins are the recommended agents
- Target body mass index is 18.5–24.9 kg/m^2

- Aspirin 75–162 mg/d
- Aerobic exercise for 30 min on most days of the week

Vaccinations
- Hepatitis B, influenza, tetanus, and pneumococcal vaccines

Medications to Avoid
- Meperidine, fleets enemas, milk of magnesia, magnesium citrate, magnesium–aluminum antacids, nitrofurantoin, NSAIDs, COX-2 inhibitors, and caution with digoxin or antiarrhythmics

Indications for Initiation of Dialysis
- Estimated GFR < 10 mL/min/1.73 m^2, uremia, unexplained weight loss, malnutrition, or decline in functioning, intractable fluid overload, refractory hypertension, and hyperkalemia, hyperphosphatemia, or metabolic acidosis refractory to treatment

Adapted from KDOQI guidelines at www.kidney.org/professionals/kdoqi/index.cfm and the KDIGO guidelines available at www.kdigo.org.

NEPHROTIC SYNDROME

Diagnostic criteria: proteinuria ≥3–3.5 g/24 hr; albumin <2.5 g/dL; peripheral edema

Associated conditions: hyperlipidemia and hypercoagulable state

Table 16-5 Etiologies of Nephrotic Syndrome in Adults

Primary (idiopathic)	Medications	Infections
• Minimal change disease • Membranous nephropathy • Focal segmental glomerulosclerosis	• Antimicrobial agents • Captopril • Gold • Lithium • NSAIDs • Penicillamine • Tamoxifen	• Filariasis • Hepatitis B and C viruses • HIV • Malaria • Mycoplasma • Schistosomiasis • Syphilis • Toxoplasmosis
Systemic diseases • Diabetes mellitus • Amyloidosis • Systemic lupus erythematosus		
Cancer • Multiple myeloma • Lymphoma		

Adapted from Brit Med J 2008;336:1185.

Evaluation of Nephrotic Syndrome
- Urinalysis to check for hematuria/infection; urine culture; 24-hr urine for protein/CrCl
- Labs: CBC, PT, PTT, chem panel, CRP, ESR, ANA, anti-dsDNA, C3, and C4 levels, fasting glucose and lipid panel; +/– glycohemoglobin
- Serologies: HIV, HBV, and HCV
- Serum and urine electrophoresis and quantitative immunoglobulins
- Consider abdominal fat pad aspirate to evaluate for amyloidosis
- Radiology: CXR; renal ultrasound with Doppler study of renal veins to rule out clot
- Renal biopsy if etiology remains unclear

Complications of Nephrotic Syndrome
- Infection is common secondary to hypogammaglobulinemia and decreased complement activity
- Venous thromboembolism and renal vein thrombosis
- Fluid overload: ascites, pleural effusions, and increased risk of CHF
- Hyperlipidemia with eruptive xanthomata and xanthelasmata

- Increased risk of cardiovascular morbidity and mortality

Treatment
- Treat the underlying cause of nephrotic syndrome
- Diet: 2 g Na/d; fluid restrict to 1.5 L/d if Na < 125 mEq/L or marked edema
  ➤ Normal dietary protein intake
- Edema management: furosemide 40–80 mg IV +/– chlorothiazide 500 mg IV or metolazone 10 mg PO 30 min prior to furosemide; administer therapy daily–tid
  ➤ Anasarca: furosemide 40–80 mg IV bid–tid right after 25% albumin 100 mL IV
- Meds: ACEI +/– ARB; data inconclusive about the safety of combined ACEI/ARB rx
  ➤ Verapamil or diltiazem can reduce proteinuria if unable to use ACEI/ARBs
  ➤ Statins ↓ risk of cardiovascular complications and may slow progression to CKD
  ➤ Aspirin 81 mg PO daily for primary cardiovascular prevention
- Keep blood pressure 125/75 mmHg or less
- Prevention: assure that pneumococcal and influenza vaccinations are up to date
  ➤ Heparin or low-molecular weight heparin for DVT prophylaxis
  ➤ Bone mineral densitometry to screen for osteoporosis

References: Brit Med J 2008;336:1185 and Nephrology 2008;13:45.

ACID–BASE INTERPRETATION

- Acidemic or alkalemic? (normal pH 7.40)
- Is the primary problem metabolic or respiratory?
  ➤ Acidosis: $pCO_2 > 40$ = respiratory; $HCO_3 < 24$ = metabolic
  ➤ Alkalosis: $pCO_2 < 40$ = respiratory; $HCO_3 > 24$ = metabolic

Respiratory Disorders
- Consider the change in pH:
  ➤ Acute respiratory acidosis or alkalosis: $\Delta pH = 0.008 \times \Delta pCO_2$
  ➤ Chronic respiratory acidosis: $\Delta pH = 0.003 \times \Delta pCO_2$
  ➤ Chronic respiratory acidosis: $\Delta pH = 0.002 \times \Delta pCO_2$
- Also, determine the expected change in HCO_3 as evidence of an acute or chronic process:
  ➤ Acute respiratory acidosis: $0.1 \times \Delta pCO_2 = \Delta HCO_3$
  ➤ Chronic respiratory acidosis: $0.35–0.4 \times \Delta pCO_2 = \Delta HCO_3$
  ➤ Acute respiratory acidosis: $0.25 \times \Delta pCO_2 = \Delta HCO_3$
  ➤ Chronic alkalosis: $0.4 \times \Delta pCO_2 = \Delta HCO_3$
- Causes of a respiratory acidosis: exacerbations of CHF, COPD, or asthma; PE; pneumonia; oversedation; obesity-hypoventilation syndrome; chronic hypoventilation from restrictive lung disease, neuromuscular disorder, or chest wall disorders; and acute intracranial injury
- Causes of a respiratory alkalosis: early sepsis; salicylate toxicity; pregnancy; cirrhosis; panic attack; severe pain, anxiety or agitation; and pulmonary embolus

Metabolic Disorders
- For a metabolic acidosis, is there an elevated anion gap (AG) or a normal AG?
  ➤ Simplified $AG = Na - Cl - HCO_3$ (normal AG = 12 +/– 2)
    ○ Hypoalbuminemia increases AG ($AG_c = AG + [(4 - albumin) \times 2]$)
  ➤ Expected $pCO_2 = 8 + (1.5 \times HCO_3)$ +/– 2 (Winter's formula)
- If an AG disorder, is there a mixed acid–base disorder ("delta delta")?
  ○ (Calculated AG – 12) + HCO_3 = 24 +/– 2 in a **simple** AG acidosis
  ○ Delta delta > 26 = concomitant metabolic alkalosis; delta delta < 22 = concomitant non-gap metabolic acidosis

> If an AG acidosis, is there an increased osmolal gap (normal ≤ 10 mOsm/kg)?
  ○ osmolal gap = $[2 \times Na + glucose/18 + BUN/2.8 + EtOH/4.6]$ − serum osm
  ○ Increased osmolal gap with alcohol, ketones, lactate, mannitol, ethylene glycol, methanol, or isopropanol (no acidosis with isopropanol)
• Causes of a high AG metabolic acidosis (mnemonic MUDPILERS)
  M—methanol
  U—uremia
  D—diabetic ketoacidosis (or other ketoacidosis—alcoholic, starvation)
  P—paraldehyde
  I—ingestions (isoniazid, iron, or toluene)
  L—lactic acidosis
  E—ethylene glycol, ethanol
  R—rhabdomyolysis (severe)
  S—salicylates or strychnine
• Causes of a non-AG metabolic acidosis (mnemonic HARDUP)
  H—hyperalimentation and post-hypocapneic
  A—acetazolamide use
  R—renal tubular acidosis (RTA)
  D—diarrhea (chronic)
  U—ureterosigmoidostomy
  P—pancreatic fistula
  > Urine AG = $U_{Na} + U_K − U_{Cl}$; a negative value = diarrhea, and positive = RTA
• Metabolic alkalosis: calculate expected pCO_2 using $\Delta pCO_2 = 0.6 \times \Delta HCO_3$
  > Chloride-responsive metabolic alkalosis (urine chloride <10–20 mmol/L)
    ○ Vomiting; high nasogastric tube output; diuretics; and rapid correction of chronic hypercapnia (post-hypercapneic)
  > Chloride-unresponsive metabolic alkalosis (urine chloride >20 mmol/L)
    ○ Excess mineralocorticoid activity
    ○ Primary hyperaldosteronism (Conn syndrome); Cushing disease; black licorice ingestion; ectopic ACTH secretion; or secondary hyperaldosteronism (renovascular disease, malignant hypertension, CHF with diuretic therapy, cirrhosis with diuretic therapy)
    ○ Significant hypokalemia
    ○ Significant hypomagnesemia
    ○ Bartter syndrome

References: NEJM 1998;338:26 and NEJM 2002;347:43.

Section 17
Rheumatology

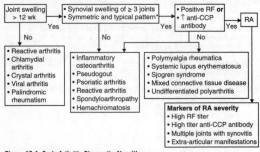

Figure 17-1 Early Arthritis Diagnostic Algorithm
RF = rheumatoid factor; CCP = cyclic citrullinated peptide.
* Typically, proximal interphalangeal, metacarpophalangeal, metatarsophalangeal, wrist, knee, elbow, or ankles involved.
Adapted from *J Rheumatol* 2005;32:203.

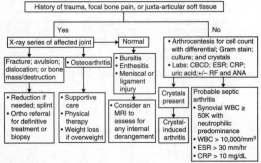

Figure 17-2 Approach to Monoarticular Arthritis
Adapted from *Am Fam Physician* 2003;68:83; *Cancer Med Assoc J* 2000;162:1577; and *JAMA* 2007;297:1478.

Table 17-1 Different Causes of Polyarthritis

Arthritis	Patient profile	History and onset	Pattern of arthritis and joints involved	X-ray findings	Supporting tests
Rheumatoid arthritis (RA)	F > M 35–50 yr	Insidious Additive ↑ AM stiffness	Symmetric; inflammatory PIP; MCP; wrist; MTP; and ankles	Joint space narrowing; bony erosions	↑ RF + α-CCP Ab ↑ CRP/ESR
UPA	F > M	Insidious Polyarthritis	Inflammatory arthritis; same joint involvement as for RA	Joint space narrowing; bony erosions	↑ CRP/ESR
Psoriatic arthritis	History of psoriasis	Insidious Additive	Inflammatory; asymmetric; DIP; PIP; knee; feet; and spine	Erosions; periostitis; osteolysis	↑ CRP/ESR; –RF; ↑ uric acid
Gout	M: 20–40 yr F: > 60 yrs	Intermittent Oligo—early Poly—later	Sudden, severe attacks; joints involved are the 1st MTP, toes; ankle, knees, and hands (late)	"Punched out" bony erosions or tophi	Synovial fluid: + monosodium urate crystals
Pseudogout	Elderly M = F	Intermittent; oligo or poly	Intermittent or chronic arthritis Knee; wrist; finger; and MTP	Chondrocalcinosis	Synovial fluid: CPPD crystals
Osteoarthritis	F > M; older patients; obesity	Insidious Additive Oligo or poly	Asymmetric; non-inflammatory; joints involved are the DIP, PIP; knee; hip; MTP; and spine	Osteophytes; joint space narrowing; subchondral sclerosis	Normal lab tests
PMR	M = F; older; caucasion	↑ AM stiffness Weight loss	Chronic and inflammatory Hip and shoulder girdles	Normal x-rays	↑ CRP/ESR; anemia; ↑ LFTs
Reactive arthritis	1–4 wk after GI/GU infection	Fever; malaise; intermittent; and extra-articular	Inflammatory; oligoarthritis; spine; knees; digits; and enthesitis	Possible sacroiliitis; periostitis; erosions; joint space narrowing	↑ CRP/ESR 40% HLA-B27-positive
SLE	F > M; young	Rash; seritis; additive	Inflammatory; joints involved are the PIP and knees	Normal x-rays of affected joints	+ ANA; ↑ CRP; ↑ ESR; ↑ dsDNA
Gonococcal arthritis	F > M, sexually active	Migratory polyarthritis	Inflammatory; wrist; knee; and tenosynovitis	Normal x-rays of affected joints	↑ CRP/ESR ↑ WBC

UPA = undifferentiated polyarthritis; PMR = polymyalgia rheumatica; SLE = systemic lupus erythematous; GI = gastrointestinal; GU = genitourinary; F = female; M = male; PIP = proximal interphalangeal; DIP = distal interphalangeal; MCP = metacarpophalangeal; MTP = metatarsophalangeal; RF = rheumatoid factor; CCP = cyclic citrullinated peptide antibody; CRP = c-reactive protein; ESR = erythrocyte sedimentation rate; CPPD = calcium pyrophosphate dehydrate; ANA = antinuclear antibody; dsDNA = double-stranded DNA; WBC = white blood count.
Adapted from *Best Pract Res Clin Rheumatol* 2006;20:653.

Table 17-2 Rheumatology Serologic Tests Reference Card

Disease	Test	Disease activity	Tests for end-organ damage and comments
Systemic lupus erythematosus (SLE)	Antinuclear antibodies (ANA)	No	Positive anti-SSA (Sjogren syndrome A) in cutaneous lupus erythematosus. Follow serial renal panel, urinalysis with micro, and complete blood count with differential.
	Anti-double-stranded DNA	Yes	
	Anti-cardiolipin/lupus anticoagulant	No	
	Anti-Smith antibodies	No	
Drug-induced LE	Antihistone antibodies*	No	Causes: carbamazepine, chlorpromazine, clindamycin, **hydralazine, isoniazid,** methyldopa, oxcarbazepine, phenytoin, and **procainamide**
Rheumatoid arthritis	Rheumatoid factor	No	X-rays of affected joints, baseline PPD and pulmonary function tests. Follow complete blood count with differential and liver panel with most therapies.
	Anti-CCP antibodies	No	
Scleroderma (CREST)	Antinuclear antibodies (ANA)	No	Anti-centromere specific for CREST syndrome. CXR, screening pulmonary function tests, blood pressure checks, renal panel, urinalysis with micro, baseline barium swallow, and EGD for any dysphagia. Echo to screen for pulmonary hypertension.
	Anticentromere	No	
	Anti-Scl70	No	
Mixed connective tissue disease	Antinuclear antibodies (ANA)	No	Renal panel, complete blood count, CK, blood pressure checks and screen for pulmonary hypertension and interstitial lung disease
	Anti-U₁-RNP (ribonucleoprotein)*	No	
Polymyositis dermatomyositis	Creatinine phosphokinase (CK)	Yes	Note: electromyogram can help to diagnose myositis. Consider search for malignancy in adult dermatomyositis. Follow creatinine phosphokinase (CK) in response to therapy.
	Anti-Jo-1 antibodies	No	
	Muscle biopsy	No	
Sjogren syndrome	Antinuclear antibodies (ANA)	No	Schirmer test for decreased tear production. Saxon test for decreased saliva production. Needs dental care and eye exams.
	Anti-SSA/Ro (Sjogren syndrome A)†	No	
	Anti-SSB/La (Sjogren syndrome B)	No	
Wegener granulomatosis	Anti-proteinase 3 antibody	Possible	Diagnosis secured with biopsy of nasopharyngeal lesion. Ear/nose/throat exam, CXR, renal panel and urinalysis +/− pulmonary function tests.
	C-antineutrophil cytoplasmic antibodies	Possible	

Disease	Test	Specificity	Sensitivity	Positive predictive value	Diagnosis
Systemic lupus erythematosus (SLE)	Antinuclear antibodies (ANA)	57%	93%	Moderate	Yes
	Anti-double-stranded DNA	97%	57%	95%	Yes
	Anti-cardiolipin/lupus anticoagulant	Yes	No	Low	No
	Anti-Smith antibodies	High	25–30%	97%	Yes
Drug-induced lupus	Antihistone antibodies*	High	95%	High	Yes
Rheumatoid arthritis	Rheumatoid factor	No	50–85%	Moderate	Yes
	Anti-CCP antibodies	90–95%	50–85%	High	No
Scleroderma (CREST)	Antinuclear antibodies (ANA)	54%	85%	High	Yes
	Anticentromere‡	99.9%	65%	High	Yes
	Anti-Scl70§	100%	20%	High	Yes
Mixed connective tissue disease	Antinuclear antibodies (ANA)	No	93%	High	Yes
	Anti-U₁-RNP (ribonucleoprotein)*	High	Moderate	High	Yes
Polymyositis dermatomyositis	Creatinine phosphokinase (CK)	No	High	Low	No
	Anti-Jo-1 antibodies	Yes	30–50%	High	Yes
	Muscle biopsy	Yes	Moderate	High	Yes
Sjogren syndrome	Antinuclear antibodies (ANA)	52%	48%	Moderate	Yes
	Anti-SSA/Ro (Sjogren syndrome)†	87%	8–70%	~40%	Yes
	Anti-SSB/La (Sjogren syndrome)	94%	16–40%	~40%	Yes
Wegener granulomatosis	Anti-proteinase 3 antibody	High	Moderate	High	Yes
	C-antineutrophil cytoplasmic antibodies	50%	95%	High	Yes

CREST = calcinosis, Raynaud phenomenon, esophageal dysmotility, sclerodactyly, and telangiectasias; Dis = disease; CCP = cyclic citrullinated peptide. *False positives from SLE. †False positive in cutaneous lupus erythematosus. ‡Anti-centromere antibodies are associated more with limited systemic sclerosis (CREST syndrome). §Anti-Scl70 is associated more with systemic sclerosis. Adapted from *South Med J* 2005;98:185.

VASCULITIS

Table 17-3 ANCA-Associated Small Vessel Vasculitis

Condition	Renal	Pulmonary	"Asthma"	Granulomas	ANCA type*	ANCA +
Wegener granulomatosis[†]	80%	90%	No	Yes	c-ANCA (anti-PR3)	90%
Microscopic[‡] polyangiitis	90%	50%	No	No	p-ANCA (anti-MPO)	70%
Churg-Strauss syndrome[§]	45%	70%	Yes	Yes	p-ANCA (anti-MPO)	50%

*Primary ANCA type seen although either c-ANCA or p-ANCA can be found in all 3 conditions.
† Presents with sinusitis, saddle-nose deformity, pulmonary infiltrates/nodules, hematuria, or pauci-immune rapidly progressive glomerulonephritis (RPGN).
‡ Presents with cough, hemoptysis, hematuria, pauci-immune RPGN, and mononeuritis multiplex.
§ Presents with eosinophilia, "asthma," neuropathy, transient lung infiltrates, coronary arteritis, and myocarditis.
Adapted from *NEJM* 1997;337:1512.

Table 17-4 Medium- and Large-Vessel Primary Vasculitis in Adults

Condition	Vessels affected	Clinical features	Diagnostic testing
Large-vessel vasculitis			
Takayasu arteritis	Aorta and its branches	"Pulseless disease" Asians; young women; fever; weight loss; limb claudication; unequal arm pulses; renovascular hypertension	• Aortogram with stenosis or occlusion of branches off aorta • Elevated ESR/CRP
Giant cell arteritis	Temporal artery and its branches	HA; jaw claudication; monocular visual loss; temporal artery tenderness; age > 50 yr	• Elevated ESR • + temporal artery biopsy
Medium-vessel vasculitis			
Polyarteritis nodosa	Medium-sized arteries	30% HBV+; fever; weight loss; myalgias; hypertension; renal failure; mononeuritis multiplex; abdominal pain	• "Beaded vessels" on mesenteric angiogram • + sural nerve biopsy • ↑ ESR and WBC
Primary CNS vasculitis	Small–medium arteries	HA; confusion; disorientation; bulbar palsies; weakness; or seizures	• Cerebral angiogram with "beaded vessels" • Brain biopsy with vasculitis

Adapted from *Curr Opin Rheum* 2006;18:1; *NEJM* 2003;349:160; *JAMA* 2002;288:1632; and *Arth Rheum* 1990;33:1065, 1129.

INDEX